THE EASY ANTI-INFLAMMATORY DIET

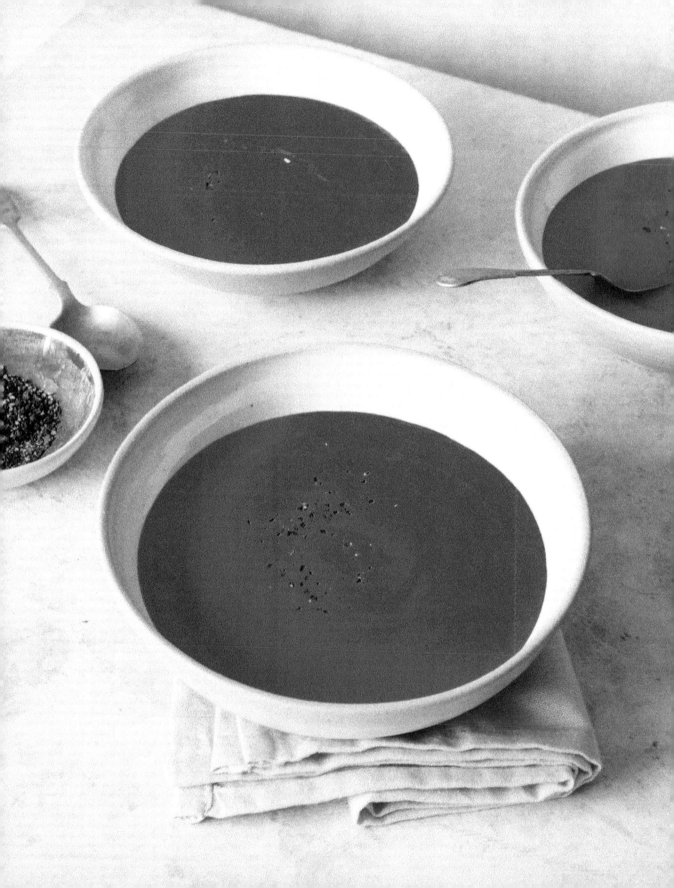

the easy ANTI-INFLAMMATORY diet

Fast and Simple Recipes for the 15 Best Anti-Inflammatory Foods

Karen Frazier

Foreword by Lulu Cook, RDN

ROCKRIDGE PRESS

For general information on our other products and services or to obtain technical support, please contact our Customer Care Department within the U.S. at (866) 744-2665, or outside the U.S. at (510) 253-0500.

Rockridge Press publishes its books in a variety of electronic and print formats. Some content that appears in print may not be available in electronic books, and vice versa.

TRADEMARKS: Rockridge Press and the Rockridge Press logo are trademarks or registered trademarks of Callisto Media Inc. and/or its affiliates, in the United States and other countries, and may not be used without written permission. All other trademarks are the property of their respective owners. Rockridge Press is not associated with any product or vendor mentioned in this book.

Cover Photography: Nat + Cody Gantz © 2017 Interior Photography: Nadine Greeff, p.ii; 82, 96, 114, 144, 156; Nat + Cody Gantz, p.vi; Ali Harper/Stocksy, p.xii; Ina Peters/Stocksy, p.24; Nataša Mandić/ Stocksy, p.38; Darren Muir/Stocksy, p.50; Jeff Wasserman/Stocksy, p.64; Ivan Solis/Stocksy, p.132.

Recipe icon Photography: Broccoli, Kale, Spinach, Tomato, Blueberries, Salmon, Almonds, Cinnamon, Garlic, Ginger, Rosemary, Turmeric, Olives, Green tea: Nat + Cody Gantz © 2017

ISBN: Print 978-1-62315-938-2 | eBook 978-1-62315-939-9

R2

For my friend Kathleen Marshall, whose life with a chronic and painful inflammatory condition is lived with kindness, compassion, and dignity that is an inspiration to me and everyone else who knows her.

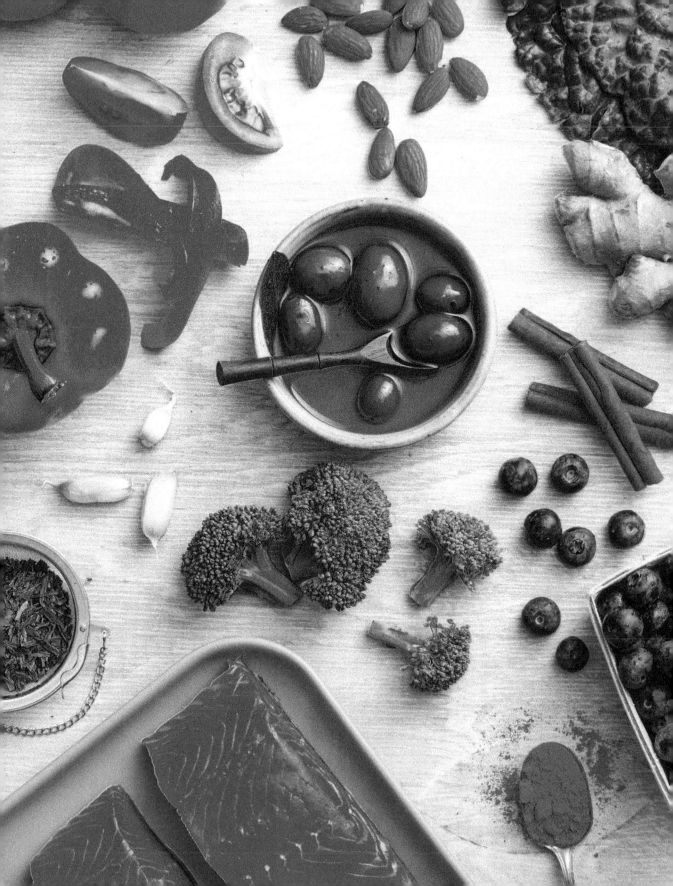

Contents

Foreword

IMAGINE HEADING HOME IN THE EVENING AFTER A FULL, BUSY DAY.
The fridge is a bit bare by this point in the week, and all the members of the household have different food preferences. You have the intention to eat in a way that will move you toward vibrant good health and reduced chronic inflammation, but you're not always sure what the best choices are. Maybe you're actively managing an autoimmune condition, or perhaps you just sense your entire system is too revved up and what you really need is an anti-inflammatory approach. But it's been a hectic day, and everybody is hungry and maybe a bit cranky. What happens next? All too often, our good intentions can sink beneath the seemingly conflicting demands of wanting meals that are affordable, convenient, fast, and, most of all, enticing. At that point, we may swing by the drive-through or tear the plastic off a package of something and throw it in the microwave, all with a feeling that we could have done better.

It doesn't have to be this way! In *The Easy Anti-Inflammatory Diet*, Karen Frazier provides simple, speedy, tempting recipes that come together quickly and are easy to customize. She explains the basics of inflammation, why it matters, and how damaging it can be to our energy and health. She also outlines what makes for successful anti-inflammatory eating—which ingredients to choose more often and which to cut back on—and she provides expert guidance on making these recipes your own as you continue to recover from chronic inflammation. While Karen incorporates plenty of fun and specialty "superfoods" (such as chia seeds and coconut oil), the recipes here are based on 15 key anti-inflammatory ingredients that are equally powerful and commonly available. And she shows you how to pull them together into inflammation-fighting, mouthwatering meals you'll enjoy.

As a registered dietitian, I work with people who want to shift their diets using anti-inflammatory principles, and I know how important it is to prepare foods at home when this is your goal. You can take charge of your health, personalize meals to meet your preferences or food allergy needs, and save money by cooking at home more. I have also heard from clients regularly that time and a lack of confidence can be obstacles in making that switch, and I am delighted to recommend this book to the people I work with—folks who are busy yet committed and who need an anti-inflammatory solution that works for their lifestyle.

When we choose to cook healthy, nourishing meals at home, food becomes a part of how we take care of ourselves and those we love. Sometimes, it can seem almost impossible to balance all those different aspects of our meal choices, and this book will help you achieve that balance—deliciously!

Lulu Cook, RDN
co-author of *The Complete Anti-Inflammatory Diet for Beginners*

P.S. Be sure to try the Blueberry, Chocolate, and Turmeric Smoothie (page 27)!

Introduction

INFLAMMATION IS NOT NECESSARILY A BAD THING. Your immune system causes inflammation in response to an injury or the presence of foreign pathogens as a way to fight off illness and heal. However, when inflammation becomes systemic and chronic, it can wreak havoc.

I know this from firsthand experience, having spent more than 25 years in a state of chronic, systemic inflammation. I was in constant pain, which was often severe. I suffered regular, recurrent migraines. My sleep quality was poor. My energy level was virtually nonexistent. I never woke feeling refreshed after a night of sleep. Instead, my body creaked and groaned, and some days it felt as if even my hair hurt.

About 10 years ago, I visited a new health care provider. She sent me for labs, including a blood test for C-reactive protein, which measures levels of inflammation. I was off the charts. It turns out I was inflamed. I am one of those people who, once I know something, can't let it go until I completely understand it. So I started researching inflammation and began making dietary changes based on what I'd learned. I noticed within a few weeks how much better I felt, and so I studied more, continued to tweak my diet, and continued to improve.

Today I am 51 years old, and I feel better than I did when I was 30. I'm energetic, I sleep well, I dance three to five times per week, and I'm active. My husband and I just finished remodeling three bathrooms—by ourselves, without the help of a contractor. It's not something I could have done even 10 years ago because I was so hobbled by inflammation.

Eating an anti-inflammatory diet–one customized for my needs–has been nothing short of life-changing. Along with helping me feel much better, become more engaged in my life, and, generally, feel more alive, it's also set me on my life's path–helping others to find the best way of eating so they, too, can optimize their health using nutritional solutions while eating fresh, flavorful foods.

It is my desire that this cookbook helps set you on a path where you, too, discover your best way to eat to feel vibrant, energetic, and pain free. This cookbook offers a basic anti-inflammatory plan based on what many experts suggest are key anti-inflammatory foods, and it avoids foods that contribute to inflammation. Because every body is different, it also offers advice to customize the plan, helping you find any personal inflammatory triggers and avoid them (for me, it's dairy and gluten; for others it may be something else).

Cooking is my livelihood and one of my life's passions, so I spend many happy hours in the kitchen puttering and testing. I'm also realistic enough to realize some people lack the time or energy to spend much time cooking or just don't share my passion. With that in mind, I designed simple, quick recipes that require minimal prep or cleanup. All recipes take fewer than 30 minutes and have five or fewer main ingredients (not including pantry staples). The recipes are easy to follow and don't require any specialized equipment, ingredients, or techniques. Each features at least one of 15 key anti-inflammatory ingredients as well as one or more secondary anti-inflammatory ingredients. The recipes also eliminate ingredients that contribute to inflammation and offer substitutions for foods that may be your personal triggers.

I'm excited to be a part of your personal path to healing.

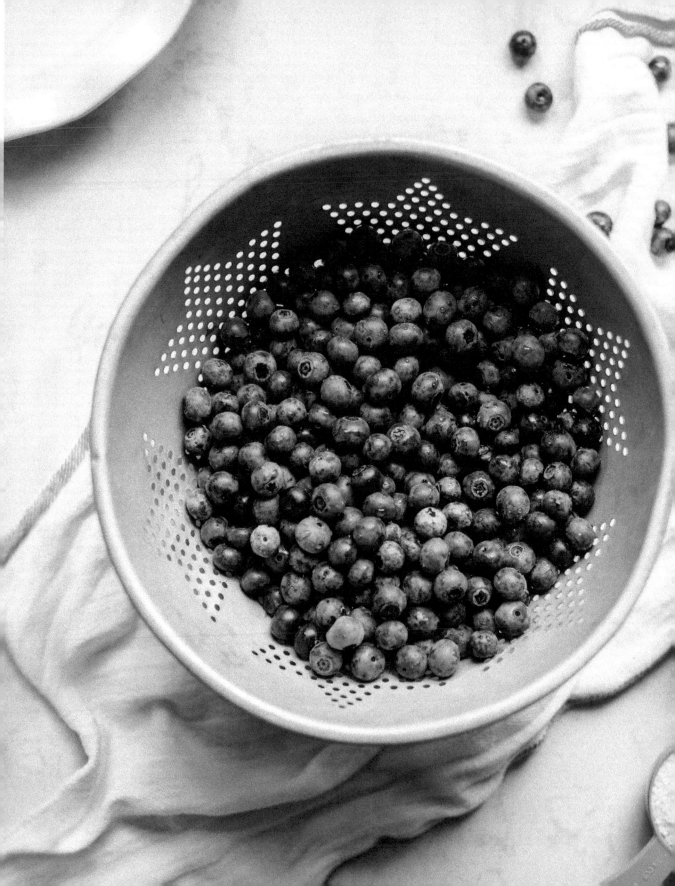

1

ANTI-INFLAMMATORY
FOODS

If you've ever injured yourself or been ill, you've experienced inflammation. According to the United States National Library of Medicine, inflammation, at its most basic, is "the body's immune system response to stimulus." In other words, it's what your body does when something that may be harmful happens.

How that occurs in your body depends on the stimulus. For example, if you get a splinter in your finger, it will become red and swollen as the body sends inflammatory cells to the area to fight potential infection and heal the injury. When foreign bacteria or viruses enter your bloodstream, the inflammatory response may result in fever, aches, and pains.

A Widespread Problem

When you are injured or ill, your body's immune response is acute, and the inflammation serves a valuable purpose—helping your body heal. As you heal, inflammation should lessen and eventually go away. Unfortunately, this isn't always the case. In recent years, chronic inflammation has become an issue for many people; something is causing the inflammation to remain, even after the acute phase of injury or illness goes away. This persistent inflammation serves no purpose and can even be harmful.

Chronic inflammation has become widespread in the past several decades, and many experts feel it underlies multiple diseases, such as auto-immune disease, heart disease, arthritis, and many others. According to the Autoimmunity Research Foundation, this trend toward diseases based on inflammatory response can be seen in death statistics from 1900 versus those from 1997. In 1900, the leading causes of death were infectious diseases, such as tuberculosis, pneumonia, and diarrhea, while in 1997 the leading causes of death were chronic inflammatory diseases including heart disease, cancer, and stroke. The Foundation also notes that in 2000, about 45 percent of the population had some sort of chronic inflammatory disease, and 21 percent had multiple chronic conditions. Those statistics are projected to continue to increase through 2030 and beyond. That's a lot of sick people.

CAUSES OF CHRONIC INFLAMMATION

Medical science is seeking to discover the roots of chronic inflammation, and according to the Autoimmunity Research Foundation, several potential causes exist. While information is based on observational studies in which researchers can find correlation, it's important to note correlation does not equal causation. This means that while causes are suggested by the studies, there isn't an abso-lutely proven concrete link between causes and outcomes. This uncertainty is inherent in epidemiological studies, but they can still supply information for the best hypotheses based on large groups of study participants.

Suggested causes for widespread chronic inflammation include:

- Antibiotic overuse and misuse (including in the food supply and through prescribed medications)
- Dietary factors (processed foods, unbalanced essential fatty acids, and chemical additives, among others)

- Environmental factors (endocrine disrupters and pesticides, among others)
- Use of substances (medications) that suppress immune responses, such as anti-inflammatories, antibacterial agents, and corticosteroids

In addition, *Medical News Today* (MNT) notes other factors that may play a role in chronic inflammation, including:

- Autoimmune diseases
- Obesity
- Poor sleep quality and sleep deprivation

Chronic Inflammatory Diseases

As research continues, a number of diseases have been linked to chronic inflammation. The following list comprises some, but not all, of the diseases, as the list is long.

AUTOINFLAMMATORY DISEASE

According to the National Institutes of Health's (NIH) National Institute of Arthritis and Musculoskeletal and Skin Diseases (NIAMS), autoinflammatory disease is a relatively new category that is different than autoimmune disease, although the names are quite similar and they share common characteristics. *Autoimmune diseases* result from the immune system attacking healthy tissue, causing chronic inflammation. The mechanism behind this response is poorly understood.

Autoinflammatory diseases present with bouts of intense, chronic inflammation that can cause symptoms such as fever and joint swelling. These diseases include:

- Behçet's disease
- Chronic Atypical Neutrophilic Dermatosis with Lipodystrophy and Elevated Temperature (CANDLE)
- Deficiency of the Interleuken-1 Receptor Agonist (DIRA)
- Familial Mediterranean Fever (FMF)
- Neonatal Onset Multisystem Inflammatory Disease (NOMID)
- Tumor Necrosis Factor Receptor-Associated Periodic Syndrome (TRAP)

AUTOIMMUNE DISEASE

NIAMS also notes that autoimmune diseases have a chronic inflammatory element to them. When your body identifies healthy tissue as a foreign invader, it attacks its own tissue. Inflammation is one of the primary signs of autoimmune disease, although, depending on the disease, other symptoms will be present as well.

There are more than 80 currently identified autoimmune diseases, according to American Autoimmune Related Diseases Association (AARDA). That's too many to list here, but a few of the common autoimmune conditions include:

- Addison's disease
- Ankylosing spondylitis
- Celiac disease
- Crohn's disease
- Endometriosis
- Fibromyalgia
- Grave's disease
- Hashimoto's disease
- Interstitial cystitis
- Juvenile arthritis

- Juvenile (type 1) diabetes
- Lupus
- Lyme disease (chronic)
- Multiple sclerosis
- Psoriasis
- Rheumatoid arthritis
- Scleroderma
- Ulcerative colitis
- Vitiligo

CARDIOVASCULAR DISEASE

The American Heart Association notes that while it isn't currently proven that inflammation is the cause of cardiovascular disease (diseases of the heart and blood vessels), it is commonly present, especially in arteries of people with this illness. Many factors associated with heart disease, such as tobacco use, high blood pressure, and high levels of "bad" cholesterol called low-density lipoprotein (LDL) also cause inflammation, so controlling these risk factors is essential in disease prevention.

TYPE 2 DIABETES AND OBESITY

An article in the May 2, 2005 issue of the *Journal of Clinical Investigation* examined the correlation between type 2 (adult onset) diabetes, inflammation, and stress, and found a close link between inflammation and type 2 diabetes, mostly centered on obesity. According to this line of research, obesity triggers a cascade of chemical responses in the body that results in widespread inflammation, and this inflammation leads to metabolic disorders such as type 2 diabetes.

Medical and Lifestyle Interventions

If you've ever suffered an acute injury, you've probably treated the inflammation (swelling, pain, immobility, and loss of function) with rest, ice, compression, and elevation (RICE), anti-inflammatory medications, and, as the inflammation goes down, heat therapy. But what about chronic inflammation?

NSAIDS

Some health experts recommend nonsteroidal anti-inflammatory drugs (NSAIDs), such as ibuprofen or naproxen sodium (Aleve), for treating inflammation. As the name suggests, these substances inhibit the body's inflammatory response. However, according to the American College of Rheumatology, the medications are not without potential side effects, especially when used long term.

CORTICOSTEROIDS

Synthetic steroids, also known as corticosteroids, are also commonly used to treat acute inflammation. Delivered topically or orally, these steroids suppress your body's immune response, which, in turn, decreases inflammation. As with NSAIDs, side effects are common with corticosteroids, particularly with long-term use.

HERBAL REMEDIES

Many alternative health care practitioners and a growing body of medical doctors recommend certain herbal remedies, such as turmeric and ginger, to fight inflammation. According to natural care specialist Dr. Andrew Weil, turmeric and ginger are among the best possible natural anti-inflammatory substances, either through dietary inclusion or supplementation. Unfortunately, according to the website ScienceDaily, turmeric isn't as bioavailable as one might hope, so combining it with substances that increase its bioavailability, such as black pepper, coconut oil, or quercetin, can help your body absorb it better.

LIFESTYLE INTERVENTIONS

Health experts also recommend lifestyle interventions that can help decrease inflammation. These include stress reduction techniques, such as exercise, yoga, and meditation, better sleep (six to eight hours per night), and weight loss.

ANTI-INFLAMMATORY DIET

The anti-inflammatory diet is a relatively new concept, and research is ongoing. However, a review in the December 2010 issue of *Nutrition in Clinical Practice* notes an anti-inflammatory eating pattern similar to the Mediterranean diet, which balances the ratio of essential fatty acids (omega-3 to omega-6 fatty acids) and consists mostly of fresh fruits, vegetables, legumes, and whole grains while minimizing saturated fats (such as fats from meat) and maximizing monounsaturated fats (such as olive oil), controls inflammation far better than the standard Western diet.

While the recipes and interventions in this book are a good start, it's important to talk to your primary health-care provider about targeted strategies for fighting inflammation. Due to the potential side effects, never self-medicate chronic inflammation with over-the-counter NSAIDs for more than a day or two. Instead, work closely with your physician or other qualified health-care provider to determine the best treatments.

You Are What You Eat

Throughout my life, I've experienced the direct effects of various nutritional approaches to managing my conditions. When I ate junk, I felt cruddy. When I ate lots of sugar, I felt sluggish. When I ate foods that didn't work well with my body's needs, my body let me know it. When I ate nutritious foods that supported my health, I felt strong and well. Clearly there was a link between what I ate and what I felt. With that in mind, I offer the basics of a nutritional approach to control chronic inflammation.

FIGHTING INFLAMMATION THROUGH DIET

The premise behind the anti-inflammatory diet is simple: focus on foods that reduce inflammation while avoiding those that contribute to it. While simple in concept, it can be more challenging in practice.

I understand this well. We live in a society where convenience is king when it comes to the foods we select. Unfortunately, many of the more convenient foods are highly processed and chock-full of inflammatory ingredients such as refined sugars and grains, chemical additives, and unhealthy fats. Still, the foods are easily available and, in some cases, taste really good, which makes the thought of giving them up difficult.

Likewise, knowing what you can eat and what you should avoid raises the degree of perceived difficulty because—let's face it—there's a lot of conflicting information available about what's "healthy" (I actually prefer the more descriptive and less marketing-friendly term "nutritious") and what's not.

The Ultimate Anti-Inflammatory Food List (page 14) is designed to help you discover at a glance which foods can help you further your goal of reducing inflammation and which may be counterproductive to your efforts. As you make food choices going forward, frequently refer to the chart. Doing so can help you make more nutritious choices that help you fight inflammation while avoiding those foods that increase it. The **Top 15 foods** (page 8) are those identified as *specifically targeted to fight inflammation*, so including even more of those in your diet can help you reduce your body's inflammatory response.

Key Ingredients

Based on current medical research, I've identified 15 key ingredients that can help fight inflammation. These ingredients appear on numerous anti-inflammatory food lists by experts in the field, including Dr. Andrew Weil and Harvard Health. The foods contain a variety of inflammation-fighting and immune-supporting ingredients, including vitamins and minerals, antioxidants, fiber, and phytonutrients.

Focusing on these 15 key ingredients makes it easier to shop, and having them on hand makes it simple to cook several recipes at once or to scan the book for a recipe based on what's in the fridge or pantry.

Every recipe here was developed contains at least one inflammation-fighting food. Although you will build your diet around these 15 ingredients, you need to include other anti-inflammatory ingredients as well. Select a variety of whole foods across a broad range of colors to meet your body's needs for micronutrients—in other words, vitamins and minerals.

THE TOP 15

Let's take a look at each key ingredient to learn how they support immunity, fight inflammation, and provide optimal nutrition.

BELL PEPPERS

Bell peppers–particularly red bell peppers–are an excellent source of antioxidants and capsaicin, both of which are fantastic inflammation fighters. Bell peppers are versatile–try them in a curry that also contains turmeric. The quercetin in the bell peppers boosts your body's absorption of anti-inflammatory curcumin. A note of caution: Bell peppers are also a nightshade. If you are sensitive to nightshades, you may need to omit them from recipes.

BROCCOLI

As a kid I didn't love broccoli, but it's since grown on me. Now I not only appreciate the flavor it brings to savory dishes, whether raw or cooked, but also its high fiber and immune-boosting antioxidants such as vitamin C. It's a cruciferous vegetable, which the Arthritis Foundation identifies as excellent for fighting inflammation.

Broccoli complements brown rice and is a confident accompaniment to lean cuts of beef, which can stand up to its strong flavor. Try stir-fried broccoli with a bit of soy sauce and some sesame seeds.

KALE

I'm from the 1980s, when kale was a garnish that nobody ate. Well, not every-body–I always ate kale. I guess I was just ahead of my time!

Kale is another cruciferous vegetable high in fiber and antioxidants. It's totally tempting in salads with a citrus and olive oil vinaigrette or cooked with garlic for an anti-inflammatory treat.

SPINACH

Popeye knew what he was doing when he popped that can of spinach, which is high in antioxidants including vitamins C and K. Spinach is one of my go-to ingredients because it is so versatile. Eat it raw in salads or enjoy it sautéed with anti-inflammatory garlic. One of my favorite spinach foods is

Spinach and Walnut Salad with Raspberry Vinaigrette (page 52). Heaven—and anti-inflammatory!

TOMATOES

Tomatoes contain lycopene, an antioxidant that may temper inflammation, according to an article in a 2010 issue of *Current Medicinal Chemistry*. It's important to note that tomatoes may cause inflammation in some people who are sensitive to nightshades (see sidebar, page 12). However, for most, tomatoes are a fabulous anti-inflammatory food. The perfect pairing for tomatoes in my mind? Garlic, basil, and olive oil. Make a simple sauce to spoon over lentils or chicken.

BLUEBERRIES

Blueberries are my favorite berry, so I'm delighted they have such a high level of antioxidants, which can help support your immune system and fight inflammation. This superfood adds a flavor burst to oatmeal, is delightful as a simple dessert, and is just the right ingredient blended with chia, cocoa powder, and almond milk for a satisfying anti-inflammatory smoothie.

SALMON AND OTHER FATTY FISH

Our bodies require a balance of essential fatty acids (omega-3 and omega-6 fatty acids) to fight inflammation properly. Omega-3 fatty acids are anti-inflammatory, while omega-6 fatty acids are pro-inflammatory. According to functional medicine specialist Chris Kresser, the ideal ratio of omega-6 fatty acids to omega-3 fatty acids is 1:1 or 2:1.

The difficulty, however, is the standard Western diet is extremely high in omega-6 fatty acids, which throws our bodies' ratio out of whack. As a result, the current ratio may be as high as 25:1, which means pro-inflammatory fatty acids greatly outweigh anti-inflammatory omega-3 fatty acids. Hence the frequent recommendation for fish oil supplementation: It's a stopgap measure to boost omega-3 fatty acids so the ratio isn't quite so unbalanced. While the science is still evolving around fish oil supplementation, it's clear that consuming fish is beneficial.

Salmon and other fatty fish (including herring, mackerel, and tuna) are excellent sources of omega-3 fatty acids, which can help boost your body's inflammation-fighting ability. Salmon is deliciously accented with greens and citrus fruits, so it's easy to make an anti-inflammatory meal with this superstar ingredient.

NUTS

The anti-inflammatory secret to nuts is their fatty acid profile. Your best bets for nuts high in omega-3 fatty acids include walnuts, macadamias, almonds, pecans, and cashews.

Nuts can be blended into desserts, sprinkled on veggies, or crushed and used to crust fish or chicken for a delightful anti-inflammatory main course. Nuts are fairly high in calories, so if weight is an issue, stick to about a handful a day to limit caloric intake and be reassured that this level of consumption has been correlated with maintaining a healthy weight range.

CINNAMON

Cinnamon, a spice that also fights inflammation, contains a substance called cinnamaldehyde, which, according to an article in the January 2008 issue of *Food and Chemical Toxicology*, inhibits inflammatory agents.

Cinnamon can be used in both sweet and savory dishes. Try it with berries, apples, or other fruits, or in the surprising combination of Shrimp with Cinnamon Sauce (page 86).

GARLIC

Garlic has long been prized for its anti-inflammatory properties, which have been proven in scientific studies, including one in the February 2014 issue of *Anticancer Agents in Medical Chemistry*. Not only does garlic fight inflammation, but it also boosts the immune system.

Garlic enhances the taste of all types of plant-based proteins, lean meats, vinaigrettes, and citrus sauces, and it pops when stir-fried with greens or broccoli. I enjoy it in chickpea hummus served with red bell peppers for dipping.

GINGER

According to the Arthritis Foundation's blog, ginger is such a powerful anti-inflammatory that it may one day replace NSAIDs as a safer alternative because it inhibits inflammation at a cellular level. One of the great things about ginger is how adaptive it is in both sweet and savory foods. Some of my favorite ways to use it include in chicken soup, and it's a perfect pair with all kinds of anti-inflammatory fruits, such as apples or pears.

ROSEMARY

Few herbs smell better than rosemary. It's fragrant, flavorful, and anti-inflammatory. According to an article in the November 2013 issue of *Planta Medica*, rosemary decreases inflammatory responses.

Rosemary goes well with chicken, lean meats, and fish. For a surprising flavor combination, toss it with strawberries and balsamic vinegar.

TURMERIC

Turmeric contains a substance called curcumin, which many studies (including one literature review in January 2013's issue of *The AAPS Journal*) have shown to be beneficial for fighting inflammation. Many people eating a typical Western diet are unfamiliar with turmeric's flavors, so they don't incorporate it into their cooking. I like fresh turmeric root in my smoothies (especially with blueberries), and it's especially good with curries, poultry, and even fish.

EXTRA-VIRGIN OLIVE OIL

The anti-inflammatory magic of extra-virgin olive oil lies in its fat profile as well as in a compound it contains called oleocanthal, which fights pro-inflammatory substances according to the Arthritis Foundation. Olive oil is also 73 percent monounsaturated fatty acids (MUFA), which are beneficial inflammation fighters.

There are numerous ways to incorporate olive oil into your anti-inflammatory diet. It's especially good mixed in vinaigrettes and tossed with dark greens, such as spinach or kale.

GREEN TEA

The University of Maryland Medical Clinic notes tea in general, and green tea specifically, as packed with antioxidants, which support immunity and fight inflammation. Its health effects have been widely documented.

Drinking green tea alone or with some honey is delightful, but you can also use green tea powder (matcha) in fruit smoothies (try it with any berry or cantaloupe).

CUSTOMIZING THE DIET

Different people react differently to certain foods. Therefore, it's important to customize this diet if you find, after following the recipes here for about 30 days, you continue to struggle with inflammation.

To customize it, I recommend eliminating all the following common triggers (from allergies and sensitivities) for 30 days and adding them back to your diet at a rate of one group per week to determine those to which you may be sensitive. During this time, keep track of your symptoms. If they recur after eating certain foods, you may be sensitive to it. See your doctor and discuss your reactions.

Nightshades: As previously mentioned, some people may be sensitive to nightshades. Foods in the nightshade category include tomatoes, tomatillos, goji berries, eggplant, bell peppers, chile peppers, and potatoes. Substitute onions, garlic, and other spices for these ingredients. For tomatoes, avoid any recipes containing them if you feel you're sensitive to nightshades.

Gluten: According to Beyond Celiac, About 1 percent of the population has an autoimmune form of gluten sensitivity called celiac disease, and another 18 million Americans may have a sensitivity to gluten called non-celiac gluten sensitivity. Gluten is a protein found in wheat, barley, rye, some oats, and foods that contain any of these ingredients. Substitute gluten-free grains, such as millet or quinoa.

Eggs: Eggs are one of the big-8 allergens. Unfortunately, for many egg dishes (like omelets), there isn't really a substitution. Skip egg-containing recipes if you are allergic. For baking, use flax eggs as a replacement. To make flax eggs, combine 1 tablespoon ground flaxseed with 2½ tablespoons water and let rest for 5 minutes to thicken. This replaces 1 egg in baking recipes.

Wheat: Wheat is another big-8 allergen, and a number of people have an immune response (different from celiac disease) to ingesting it. Substitute buckwheat or rice flour for wheat.

Dairy Products: Dairy is a common allergy. People (including me) may be allergic to the milk proteins (casein or whey), while others may be sensitive to a sugar in milk called lactose. Substitute nondairy milks, such as unsweetened almond milk or hemp milk.

Tree Nuts: Allergies to the proteins in tree nuts are also common. Tree nuts include almonds, walnuts, pecans, cashews, Brazil nuts, and macadamia nuts. If you are allergic to tree nuts, you may be able to substitute peanuts.

Peanuts: While most people consider peanuts a nut, they are actually a legume, so the allergy to a peanut protein isn't the same as the one to tree nuts. Many people are allergic to one or the other, but not both, while some people may be allergic to both. If you have an allergy to one but not the other, substitute between the groups.

Soy: Soy, another common allergen, is ubiquitous in processed foods. It's also present in whole foods and minimally processed healthy plant-based ingredients such as edamame, tempeh, soy sauce, and miso. If allergic to soy, substitute a protein such as chicken for tofu, and replace soy sauce or miso with extra herbs and spices.

Shellfish: Shellfish, including crustaceans such as shrimp and scallops, and mollusks such as mussels and clams, are another common allergen. While some people may be allergic to both fish and shellfish, many people are allergic to one or the other. If you are allergic to only one, substitute fish for shellfish or vice versa. Otherwise, substitute tofu or chicken.

Fish: Just as some people are allergic to proteins in shellfish, others are allergic to fish, such as cod, salmon, trout, and halibut. If you are allergic to fish, substitute shellfish. If you're allergic to both, substitute tofu or chicken. Replace fish sauce and Worcestershire sauce with soy sauce.

> **A NOTE ABOUT EATING OFF PLAN**
>
> I use a guideline for my eating plan called the 90–10 guideline. If I eat on track 90 percent of the time, about 10 percent of the time I can add a few inflammatory ingredients (as long as I'm not allergic or sensitive to them), and I don't experience the effects of inflammation. Because of that, you will find a few small amounts of inflammatory ingredients in some recipes.

THE ULTIMATE ANTI-INFLAMMATORY FOOD LIST

VEGETABLES

Ingredients that May Trigger Inflammation
AVOID OR MINIMIZE

Corn • Potatoes

Ingredients that Reduce Inflammation
ENJOY

Acorn squash • Artichoke • Arugula • Asparagus • Beans, green • Beet greens • Beets • Bok choy • Broccolini • Broccoli rabe • Brussels sprouts • Butternut squash • Cabbage • Carrots • Cauliflower • Chayote • Celeriac (celery root) • Celery • Collard greens • Cucumber • Dulse • Edamame • Eggplant • Endive • Frisée • Fennel • Grape leaves • Hearts of palm • Jicama • Kohlrabi Leeks • Lettuce (all types) • Mushrooms • Mustard greens • Nopales • Nori • Okra • Onions • Parsnip • Pattypan squash • Pea pods • Pumpkin • Purslane • Rapini • Rutabaga • Scallions • Shallots • Spaghetti squash • Spinach • Sprouts • Sunchoke • Sweet potato • Swiss chard • Tomatoes, canned (sugar-free) • Tomato sauce (sugar-free) • Tomatillo • Turnip • Turnip greens • Wakame • Water chestnut • Watercress • Yam • Zucchini

15 Key Ingredients
EAT IN ABUNDANCE

BELL PEPPERS • BROCCOLI • KALE • SPINACH • TOMATOES

GRAINS AND STARCHES

Ingredients that May Trigger Inflammation
AVOID OR MINIMIZE

Baked goods (bread, cookies, donuts, pies, etc.) • Bread, white • Cereal • Flour, white • Oatmeal, instant, with sugar • Pasta • Potato starch • Rice, white • Wheat, refined

Ingredients that Reduce Inflammation
ENJOY

Amaranth • Arrowroot • Barley • Bulgur • Buckwheat • Corn • Cornstarch • Farro • Kamut • Millet • Oats, rolled • Quinoa • Rice, brown • Rye • Teff • Wheat, cracked • Wheat, whole • Wild rice

THE ULTIMATE ANTI-INFLAMMATORY FOOD LIST

FRUITS

Ingredients that May Trigger Inflammation
AVOID OR MINIMIZE

Processed juices with added sugar
Canned fruit in syrup

Ingredients that Reduce Inflammation
ENJOY

Acai • Apple • Apricot • Asian pear • Avocado • Banana • Blackberry • Blackcurrant • Blood orange • Boysenberry • Breadfruit • Canary melon • Cantaloupe • Casaba melon • Charentais (melon) • Cherry • Chokecherry • Clementine • Coconut • Cranberry • Currant • Date • Dragon fruit • Durian • Elderberry • Fig • Galia (melon) • Goji berry • Gooseberry • Grape • Grapefruit • Guava • Honeydew • Horned melon • Huckleberry • Jackfruit • Kiwi • Kumquat • Lemon • Lime • Lychee • Mandarin • Mango • Mangosteen • Marionberry • Mulberry • Nectarine • Orange • Olives • Papaya • Passionfruit • Peach • Pear • Persian melon • Persimmon • Pineapple • Plantain • Plum • Pluot • Pomegranate • Pomelo • Prickly pear • Prunes • Quince • Raisin • Raspberry • Red currant • Salmonberry • Santa Claus melon • Satsuma • Star fruit • Strawberry • Tamarind • Tangerine • Tayberry • Ugli fruit • Watermelon • Yuzu

15 Key Ingredients
EAT IN ABUNDANCE

BLUEBERRIES

THE ULTIMATE ANTI-INFLAMMATORY FOOD LIST

MEATS, POULTRY, FISH, AND PROTEINS

Ingredients that May Trigger Inflammation
AVOID OR MINIMIZE

Bacon • Beef, feedlot • Beef, New York strip • Beef, prime rib • Beef, rib eye • Bologna • Brains (all types) • Catfish, fried • Chicken, fried • Cured meats • Deli meats • Farmed seafood • Fish, fried • Foie gras • Gizzards • Ham • Heart (all types) • Hot dogs • Kidney (all types) • Lamb, rack • Lamb, rib chops • Liver (all types) • Pork, ground • Salami • Sausage • Scallops, fried • Shrimp, fried • Trout, fried • Whey protein

Ingredients that Reduce Inflammation
ENJOY

Anchovy • Bass, wild-caught • Beef, lean or very lean • Bison, lean • Catfish, wild-caught • Chicken, free-range, skinless • Clams • Cod • Duck, free-range, skinless • Eggs • Elk • Halibut • Lamb, very lean cuts • Mussels • Orange roughy • Pork, boneless top loin chop • Pork, center loin chop • Pork, rib chop • Pork, sirloin roast • Pork, tenderloin (preferably pastured) • Pork, top loin roast • Razor clams • Scallops • Shrimp • Skate • Snapper • Sturgeon, wild-caught • Tilapia, wild-caught • Turkey, free-range, skinless • Venison

15 Key Ingredients
EAT IN ABUNDANCE

SALMON (AND OTHER FATTY FISH INCLUDING TUNA, MACKEREL, SARDINES, AND TROUT)

NUTS, SEEDS, AND LEGUMES

Ingredients that Reduce Inflammation
ENJOY

Adzuki beans • Almond butter • Almonds, raw • Black beans • Brazil nuts, raw • Cashews, raw • Chia seeds • Chickpeas (garbanzo beans) • Cocoa beans (dark chocolate, cocoa powder) • Fava beans • Flaxseed • Hazelnuts, raw • Kidney beans • Lentils • Lima beans • Macadamia nuts, raw • Peanut butter • Peanuts, raw • Peas, black-eyed • Peas, green • Peas, snow • Peas, split • Peas, sugar snap • Pecans, raw • Pine nuts • Pinto beans • Pistachios, raw • Poppy seeds • Sesame seeds • Soybeans • Sunflower seeds • Walnuts, raw

15 Key Ingredients
EAT IN ABUNDANCE

NUTS

THE ULTIMATE ANTI-INFLAMMATORY FOOD LIST

VEGETABLES, HERBS, AND SPICES

Ingredients that May Trigger Inflammation
AVOID OR MINIMIZE

Garlic salt • Seasoning salt • Spice blends with sugar • Table salt

Ingredients that Reduce Inflammation
ENJOY

Allspice • Anise • Anise, star • Asafoetida • Basil • Bay leaves • Caraway • Cassia • Cayenne • Celery salt • Chamomile • Chile peppers • Chinese five-spice powder • Chipotle • Chives • Cilantro • Coriander • Cumin • Curry powder • Dill • Fennel seed • Fenugreek • Galangal • Garam masala • Herbes de Provence • Horseradish • Juniper berry • Lavender • Lemongrass • Lemon pepper • Lemon zest • Lime zest • Mace • Marjoram • Mint • Mustard powder • Mustard seed • Nutmeg • Onion powder • Orange zest • Oregano • Paprika • Parsley • Pepper (black) • Radicchio • Radish • Red pepper flakes • Rhubarb • Sage • Saffron • Salt, Himalayan pink and sea • Spearmint • Sumac • Tarragon • Thyme • Vanilla bean

15 Key Ingredients
EAT IN ABUNDANCE

CINNAMON • GARLIC • GINGER • ROSEMARY • TURMERIC

FATS AND OILS

Ingredients that May Trigger Inflammation
AVOID OR MINIMIZE

Butter • Canola oil • Corn oil • Sesame oil • Soybean oil • Hydrogenated oils • Lite olive oil • Margarine • Palm oil • Peanut oil • Safflower oil • Shortening • Sunflower oil • Vegetable oil

Ingredients that Reduce Inflammation
ENJOY

Avocado oil • Coconut oil • Macadamia oil

15 Key Ingredients
EAT IN ABUNDANCE

EXTRA-VIRGIN OLIVE OIL

THE ULTIMATE ANTI-INFLAMMATORY FOOD LIST

DAIRY AND DAIRY ALTERNATIVES

Ingredients that May Trigger Inflammation
AVOID OR MINIMIZE

Cheese, dairy (all types) • Cow's milk (all types) • Kefir, cow's milk • Goat's milk • Half-and-half • Heavy (whipping) cream • Ice cream • Nondairy creamer • Sour cream • Whipped cream

Ingredients that Reduce Inflammation
ENJOY

Almond milk, unsweetened • Coconut milk, lite, unsweetened • Coconut milk, full-fat, unsweetened • Hemp milk, unsweetened • Kefir, water • Soymilk, unsweetened • Yogurt, coconut, plain, unsweetened • Yogurt, almond, plain, unsweetened • Yogurt, dairy • Yogurt, Greek

SWEETENERS

Ingredients that May Trigger Inflammation
AVOID OR MINIMIZE

Acesulfame-K (Acesulfame potassium) • Agave nectar • Aspartame (NutraSweet) • Erythritol • Mannitol • Molasses, refined • Saccharine • Sorbitol • Sucralose (Splenda) • Sugar alcohols • Sugar, brown and powdered • Syrup, brown rice, corn, high fructose corn, maple (artificial), simple • Xylitol

Ingredients that Reduce Inflammation
ENJOY

Honey • Maple syrup, pure • Stevia

THE ULTIMATE ANTI-INFLAMMATORY FOOD LIST

CONDIMENTS

Ingredients that May
Trigger Inflammation
AVOID OR MINIMIZE

Barbecue sauce • Cocktail sauce • Ketchup • Mayonnaise (store-bought) • Vinaigrette (store-bought) • Salad dressing • Salsa, with sugar • Teriyaki sauce (store-bought)

Ingredients that Reduce
Inflammation
ENJOY

Anchovy paste • Fish sauce, sugar-free • Horseradish, prepared, sugar-free • Hot sauce, sugar-free • Mayonnaise (homemade) • Miso • Mustard, Dijon • Mustard, ground • Salsa, sugar-free • Soy sauce • Tahini • Tamari • Teriyaki sauce, sugar-free (homemade) • Tomato paste • Vinaigrette (homemade) • Vinegar, all kinds • Wasabi • Worcestershire sauce

BEVERAGES

Ingredients that May
Trigger Inflammation
AVOID OR MINIMIZE

Beer • Artificially or sugar sweetened drinks • Energy drinks • Juice, sweetened • Liquor, hard • Liqueurs • Milk, dairy • Soda, diet • Soda, regular • Soft drinks, sweetened (with sugar or artificial sweetener)

Ingredients that Reduce
Inflammation
ENJOY

Chai (with nondairy milk and no sugar) • Coffee • Kombucha • Wine (limit 4 oz.)

15 Key Ingredients
EAT IN ABUNDANCE

TEA (PARTICULARLY GREEN TEA) • WATER

Pantry Essentials

One of the best ways to stay on track with your new food regimen is to keep a well-stocked pantry filled with items you need to cook your anti-inflammatory meals. Having the important items on hand makes it easier to cook meals efficiently without extra trips to the grocery store.

Stock your pantry with the following essentials.

OILS, VINEGARS, AND CONDIMENTS

- Mustard, Dijon
- Olive oil, extra-virgin
- Soy sauce, low-sodium (or gluten-free or tamari)
- Vinegar, apple cider

HERBS AND SPICES

- Chili powder
- Cinnamon, ground
- Curry powder
- Garlic powder
- Ginger, ground
- Onion powder
- Oregano, dried
- Nutmeg, ground
- Peppercorns
- Red pepper flakes
- Rosemary, dried
- Salt, Himalayan pink or sea
- Thyme, dried
- Turmeric, ground

NUTS, SEEDS, LEGUMES, AND GRAINS

- Almond butter
- Chickpeas, canned
- Beans, black, canned
- Beans, kidney, canned
- Lentils, canned
- Peanut butter
- Quinoa
- Rice, brown, cooked
- Sesame seeds, toasted
- Sunflower seeds

CANNED ITEMS

- Broth, chicken, no salt added
- Broth, vegetable, no salt added
- Coconut milk, lite
- Red bell peppers, roasted, in oil
- Tomatoes, chopped
- Tomatoes, crushed

SUGAR, BAKING INGREDIENTS, AND FLOURS

- Arrowroot powder (or cornstarch)
- Cocoa powder, unsweetened
- Honey
- Maple syrup, pure
- Stevia
- Sugar, brown
- Vanilla extract

OTHER

- Green tea
- Milk, almond, hemp, or rice, unsweetened

Time-Saving Tips

The quick (30-minute) recipes in this book use five or fewer main ingredients (aside from pantry staples) and provide the easiest way to enjoy an anti-inflammatory diet. But there are ways to make cooking at home even easier; a little planning and preparation can help you stay on track and feel better in less time.

Plan a week at a time. When my kids were small, I planned our weekly meals (sometimes a month's worth) every weekend. Based on my plan, I made a shopping list (categorized by food type or location in the grocery store) so I could get in and out quickly.

Cook once, eat twice. This is my all-time favorite time-saving tip that you'll see in every cookbook I've written. I routinely cook double batches so I can make two meals at once. We eat that meal one night and the leftovers another day, or I freeze the leftovers for the next week.

Get creative with leftovers. Another thing I recommend is to find multiple uses for a food you've prepared. For example, if I cook a chicken for a meal, I may cook extra and freeze it to use in a soup later in the week. It's a variation of cooking once, eating twice, and it saves a lot of time.

Make liberal use of prepared veggies. The grocery store salad bar is your friend when you want to save time, as are any containers of prechopped veggies. When I'm in a hurry, I may buy prechopped onions and carrots. As soon as I get home, I'm ready to go without having to prep foods. This is great for busy weeknights.

When you just don't have time, use a slow cooker. Many recipes in this book can easily be adapted for the slow cooker. While that increases the cooking time to eight hours, you just toss the ingredients (great for chilis, soups, and stews) in the slow cooker, set it on low heat, and come home to a hot meal.

Prep on the weekends. If I have a super-busy week coming up, after I plan my meals and shop, I also prep and cook my meals to freeze or refrigerate so I can pull them out as the week progresses. In a Sunday afternoon, you can prep meals for the entire week.

Frozen veggies and fruits save time. Frozen vegetables and fruits tend to be nutritious because they are flash frozen at the peak of ripeness, and they are usually prechopped as well. This is a great time saver when you're super busy.

Consider getting help with chopping. Want to chop stuff super-fast? A food processor, a pull chopper, a spiralizer, or a mandoline all make quick work of chopping veggies and herbs. I can't live without my food processor. Well, I can. But I don't want to.

Only chop herbs once. Another of my little secrets is this: I chop a bunch of herbs (usually in my food processor) and freeze them in ice cube trays in 1 tablespoon extra-virgin olive oil. Once frozen, I pop them out of the trays and store them in labeled resealable bags. When it's time to cook, I just toss them in the pot.

Pre-chop fruits and veggies. Spend 30 minutes on a Sunday doing fruit and veggie prep for the week. Wash 'em, peel 'em, chop 'em, and freeze or refrigerate them and toss them in your food when you're ready to cook.

About the Recipes

All recipes in this book use fewer than five ingredients (not counting pantry staples), and take only 30 minutes total (prep plus cooking time) to prepare. They are organized by course, and each calls out a key ingredient as well as other supporting anti-inflammatory ingredients.

The recipes contain inexpensive, commonly available ingredients and don't require any special equipment or techniques. Many recipes can be cooked in a single pot, which minimizes the cleanup. There are also helpful tips on how to prepare or work with certain ingredients, make substitutions for common allergens, vary the recipe, or refrigerate and freeze leftovers.

Each recipe contains labels that can help you plan your meals. The recipe labels are as follows:

Dairy-Free: contains no dairy products from cows or goats, although they may contain alternative, plant-based dairy sources

Gluten-Free: completely gluten-free and safe to consume if you're gluten sensitive or have celiac disease

Nut-Free: contains no peanuts, tree nuts, or nut butters; perfect for people with nut allergies

One Pot: cooks in a single pot or pan; cleanup is minimal

Vegan: contains no animal products, including honey

Vegetarian: contains no meat, poultry, or fish, but may contain eggs, dairy, or honey

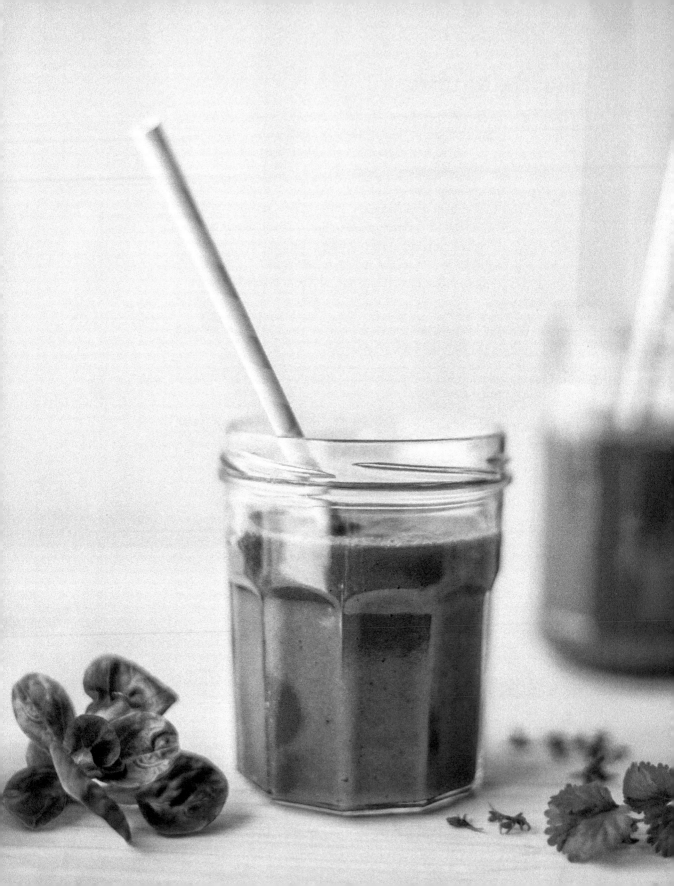

2

SMOOTHIES & BREAKFASTS

‹‹ Green Smoothie, page 26

SPINACH

GINGER

DAIRY-FREE
GLUTEN-FREE
NUT-FREE
ONE POT
VEGAN

Green Smoothie

SERVES 2 / PREP TIME 5 MINUTES

Smoothies are a quick way to pack in anti-inflammatory ingredients, and this version is loaded with nutritious spinach. Adding some fruit helps add a touch of sweetness without sugar overload.

3 CUPS BABY SPINACH

¼ CUP CILANTRO LEAVES

2 PEARS, PEELED, CORED, AND CHOPPED

3 CUPS UNSWEETENED APPLE JUICE

1 TABLESPOON GRATED GINGER

1 CUP CRUSHED ICE

In a blender, combine the spinach, cilantro, pears, apple juice, ginger, and ice. Blend until smooth.

PER SERVING Calories: 308; Total Fat: <1g; Total Carbs: 77g; Sugar: 61g; Fiber: 8g; Protein: 2g; Sodium: 50mg

Blueberry, Chocolate, and Turmeric Smoothie

SERVES 2 / PREP TIME 5 MINUTES

This is one of my favorite smoothies. I like to use frozen wild blueberries (I think they taste better than cultivated blueberries), and, whenever possible, I use fresh turmeric. You can, however, substitute 1 teaspoon ground turmeric. I find fresh turmeric's flavor relatively mild with a nice peppery bite that complements the other ingredients.

2 CUPS UNSWEETENED ALMOND MILK

1 CUP FROZEN WILD BLUEBERRIES

2 TABLESPOONS COCOA POWDER

1 TO 2 PACKETS STEVIA, OR TO TASTE

1 (1-INCH) PIECE FRESH TURMERIC, PEELED

1 CUP CRUSHED ICE

In a blender, combine the almond milk, blueberries, cocoa powder, stevia, turmeric, and ice. Blend until smooth.

SUBSTITUTION TIP: If you are allergic to tree nuts, replace the almond milk with either unsweetened hemp milk or plain rice milk.

PER SERVING Calories: 97; Total Fat: 5g; Total Carbs: 16g; Sugar: 7g; Fiber: 5g; Protein: 3g; Sodium: 182mg

CINNAMON

KALE

DAIRY-FREE
GLUTEN-FREE
ONE POT
VEGAN

Kale and Banana Smoothie

SERVES 2 / PREP TIME 5 MINUTES

Green smoothies have recently entered the popular consciousness as a great way to add green veggies into your diet. I've long used fruit and green smoothies in my house as a "sneak attack" when teenage boys (now adults) used to fight greens with all their might. They were none the wiser.

2 CUPS UNSWEETENED ALMOND MILK

2 CUPS KALE, STEMMED, LEAVES CHOPPED

2 BANANAS, PEELED

1 TO 2 PACKETS STEVIA, OR TO TASTE

1 TEASPOON GROUND CINNAMON

1 CUP CRUSHED ICE

In a blender, combine the almond milk, kale, bananas, stevia, cinnamon, and ice. Blend until smooth.

SUBSTITUTION TIP: If you are allergic to tree nuts, replace the almond milk with either unsweetened hemp milk or plain rice milk. If you don't think the banana covers the kale well enough (if your plan is sneaking in greens), add 1 cup brightly colored berries, such as blueberries.

PER SERVING Calories: 181; Total Fat: 4g; Total Carbs: 37g; Sugar: 15g; Fiber: 6g; Protein: 4g; Sodium: 210mg

Green Tea and Pear Smoothie

SERVES 2 / PREP TIME 5 MINUTES

While you're certainly welcome to simply brew and drink a cup of green tea, adding it to a smoothie is a great way to get some green tea goodness even if you're not a tea drinker. Use decaffeinated tea if you wish. The pear and ginger support the delicate flavor of the tea in this surprising smoothie combination.

2 CUPS STRONGLY BREWED GREEN TEA

2 PEARS, PEELED, CORED, AND CHOPPED

2 TABLESPOONS HONEY

1 (1-INCH) PIECE FRESH GINGER, PEELED AND ROUGHLY CHOPPED, OR 1 TEASPOON GROUND GINGER

1 CUP UNSWEETENED ALMOND MILK

1 CUP CRUSHED ICE

In a blender, combine the green tea, pears, honey, ginger, almond milk, and ice. Blend until smooth.

SUBSTITUTION TIP: If you are allergic to tree nuts, replace the almond milk with either unsweetened hemp milk or plain rice milk. If you don't feel like brewing tea, use 1 tablespoon matcha powder, which is a green tea powder available online and in many grocery stores. If you use matcha powder, increase the almond milk to 2 cups.

PER SERVING Calories: 208; Total Fat: 2g; Total Carbs: 51g; Sugar: 38g; Fiber: 7g; Protein: 1g; Sodium: 94mg

GINGER

GREEN TEA

DAIRY-FREE
GLUTEN-FREE
ONE POT
VEGETARIAN

BLUEBERRIES

WALNUTS

GLUTEN-FREE
ONE POT
VEGETARIAN

Yogurt, Berry, and Walnut Parfait

SERVES 2 / PREP TIME 10 MINUTES

Layer this in a parfait glass or mix it together in a bowl. I typically go with the bowl unless I'm trying to impress guests—it's quicker and easier. This is a simple, filling breakfast that also makes a great midday snack.

2 CUPS PLAIN UNSWEETENED YOGURT, OR PLAIN UNSWEETENED COCONUT YOGURT OR ALMOND YOGURT

2 TABLESPOONS HONEY

1 CUP FRESH BLUEBERRIES

1 CUP FRESH RASPBERRIES

½ CUP WALNUT PIECES

1. In a medium bowl, whisk the yogurt and honey. Spoon into 2 serving bowls.

2. Top each with ½ cup blueberries, ½ cup raspberries, and ¼ cup walnut pieces.

PER SERVING Calories: 505; Total Fat: 22g; Total Carbs: 56g; Sugar: 45g; Fiber: 8g; Protein: 23g; Sodium: 174mg

Ginger-Berry Smoothie

SERVES 2 / PREP TIME 10 MINUTES

I prefer the flavor of fresh ginger in my smoothies; if you don't, substitute 1 teaspoon ground ginger. Make this nut free by replacing the almond milk with unsweetened rice milk or hemp milk.

2 CUPS FRESH BLACKBERRIES

2 CUPS UNSWEETENED ALMOND MILK

1 TO 2 PACKETS STEVIA, OR TO TASTE

1 (1-INCH) PIECE FRESH GINGER, PEELED AND ROUGHLY CHOPPED

2 CUPS CRUSHED ICE

In a blender, combine the blackberries, almond milk, stevia, ginger, and ice. Blend until smooth.

INGREDIENT TIP: To peel fresh ginger just cut off a piece and use a vegetable peeler to remove the outer layer.

PER SERVING Calories: 95; Total Fat: 3g; Total Carbs: 16g; Sugar: 7g; Fiber: 9g; Protein: 3g; Sodium: 152mg

GINGER

DAIRY-FREE
GLUTEN-FREE
ONE POT
VEGAN

GREEN TEA

TURMERIC

DAIRY-FREE
GLUTEN-FREE
ONE POT
VEGETARIAN

Turmeric and Green Tea Mango Smoothie

SERVES 2 / PREP TIME 5 MINUTES

While this recipe calls for powdered turmeric that you can find in your spice aisle, if you can find fresh turmeric, it's a great substitution here. It's usually in the produce aisle near the ginger, but turmeric roots are smaller and resemble grubs. Substitute 1 (1-inch) fresh turmeric root, peeled and chopped, for the dried turmeric if you use fresh.

2 CUPS CUBED MANGO

2 TEASPOONS TURMERIC POWDER

2 TABLESPOONS MATCHA (GREEN TEA) POWDER

2 CUPS ALMOND MILK

2 TABLESPOONS HONEY

1 CUP CRUSHED ICE

In a blender, combine the mango, turmeric, matcha, almond milk, honey, and ice. Blend until smooth.

PER SERVING Calories: 285; Total Fat: 3g; Total Carbs: 68g; Sugar: 63g; Fiber: 6g; Protein: 4g; Sodium: 94mg

Green Tea and Ginger Shake

SERVES 2 / PREP TIME 5 MINUTES

This is a quick and easy recipe for an anti-inflammatory milkshake. It only takes a minute or two, and you can have a little bit of sweet with your anti-inflammatory ingredients.

2 TABLESPOONS GRATED GINGER

2 TABLESPOONS HONEY

2 TABLESPOONS MATCHA (GREEN TEA) POWDER

2 SCOOPS LOW-FAT VANILLA ICE CREAM

2 CUPS SKIM MILK

In a blender, combine the ginger, honey, matcha, ice cream, and milk. Blend until smooth.

SUBSTITUTION TIP: To make this dairy free, you can use any nondairy milk and any nondairy ice cream, such as almond milk and almond milk ice cream.

PER SERVING Calories: 340; Total Fat: 7g; Total Carbs: 56g; Sugar: 50g; Fiber: 2g; Protein: 11g; Sodium: 186mg

GINGER

GREEN TEA

DAIRY-FREE
NUT-FREE

CINNAMON

DAIRY-FREE
GLUTEN-FREE
ONE POT
VEGAN

Oatmeal and Cinnamon with Dried Cranberries

SERVES 2 / PREP TIME 5 MINUTES / COOK TIME 8 MINUTES

Use old-fashioned oats here—not quick oats or instant oatmeal, which have smaller pieces. The texture is better and the cook time isn't that much longer—it's worth it. Replace the dried cranberries with other fruits, such as dried apples or apricots, if you prefer. If you don't consume tree nuts, replace the almond milk with either 1 cup water or unsweetened rice milk or hemp milk.

1 CUP WATER

1 CUP ALMOND MILK

PINCH SEA SALT

1 CUP OLD-FASHIONED OATS

½ CUP DRIED CRANBERRIES

1 TEASPOON GROUND CINNAMON

1. In a medium saucepan over high heat, bring the water, almond milk, and salt to a boil.

2. Stir in the oats, cranberries, and cinnamon. Reduce the heat to medium and cook for 5 minutes, stirring occasionally.

3. Remove the oatmeal from the heat. Cover the pot and let it stand for 3 minutes. Stir before serving.

PER SERVING Calories: 101; Total Fat: 2g; Total Carbs: 18g; Sugar: 1g; Fiber: 4g; Protein: 3g; Sodium: 126mg

Spinach Frittata

SERVES 4 / PREP TIME 10 MINUTES / COOK TIME 12 MINUTES

If you don't consume dairy products, omit the cheese in this recipe. While cheeses (and other dairy products) are inflammatory, this dish only includes a small amount, so it shouldn't have a huge inflammatory effect unless you are allergic. I can eat frittatas for breakfast, lunch, or dinner. Leftovers refrigerate or freeze well.

2 TABLESPOONS EXTRA-VIRGIN OLIVE OIL

2 CUPS FRESH BABY SPINACH

8 EGGS, BEATEN

1 TEASPOON GARLIC POWDER

½ TEASPOON SEA SALT

⅛ TEASPOON FRESHLY GROUND BLACK PEPPER

2 TABLESPOONS GRATED PARMESAN CHEESE

1. Preheat the broiler to high.

2. In a large ovenproof skillet (well-seasoned cast iron works well) over medium-high heat, heat the olive oil until it shimmers.

3. Add the spinach and cook for about 3 minutes, stirring occasionally.

4. In a medium bowl, whisk the eggs, garlic powder, salt, and pepper. Carefully pour the egg mixture over the spinach and cook the eggs for about 3 minutes until they begin to set around the edges.

5. Using a rubber spatula, gently pull the eggs away from the edges of the pan. Tilt the pan to let the uncooked egg flow into the edges. Cook for 2 to 3 minutes until the edges set.

6. Sprinkle with the Parmesan cheese and put the skillet under the broiler. Broil for about 3 minutes until the top puffs.

7. Cut into wedges to serve.

STORAGE TIP: You can freeze frittata wedges in resealable bags for up to 3 months. They will also hold in the fridge for 4 days.

PER SERVING Calories: 203; Total Fat: 17g; Total Carbs: 2g; Sugar: <1g; Fiber: <1g; Protein: 13g; Sodium: 402mg

EXTRA-VIRGIN OLIVE OIL

GARLIC

SPINACH

GLUTEN-FREE
NUT-FREE
VEGETARIAN

**EXTRA-VIRGIN
OLIVE OIL**

**RED BELL
PEPPER**

DAIRY-FREE

GLUTEN-FREE

NUT-FREE

VEGETARIAN

Mushroom and Bell Pepper Omelet

SERVES 2 / PREP TIME 10 MINUTES / COOK TIME 10 MINUTES

I love veggies in my omelet. Red bell peppers go well with eggs and mushrooms, making this a flavorful and hearty breakfast choice. Many local grocery stores sell prechopped bell peppers, a great option if you want to save time. You can also buy presliced mushrooms.

**2 TABLESPOONS EXTRA-VIRGIN
OLIVE OIL**

1 RED BELL PEPPER, SLICED

1 CUP MUSHROOMS, SLICED

6 EGGS, BEATEN

½ TEASPOON SEA SALT

**⅛ TEASPOON FRESHLY GROUND
BLACK PEPPER**

1. In a large nonstick skillet over medium-high heat, heat the olive oil until it shimmers.

2. Add the red bell pepper and mushrooms. Cook for about 4 minutes, stirring occasionally, until soft.

3. In a medium bowl, whisk the eggs, salt, and pepper. Pour the eggs over the vegetables and cook for about 3 minutes without stirring until the eggs begin to set around the edges.

4. Using a rubber spatula, gently pull the eggs away from the edges of the pan. Tilt the pan so the uncooked egg can flow to the edges. Cook for 2 to 3 minutes until the eggs are set at the edges and the center.

5. Using a spatula, fold the omelet in half. Cut into wedges to serve.

INGREDIENT TIP: To clean mushrooms (if you don't buy them presliced), don't run water over them. They are like little sponges that will soak it all up. Instead, use a soft brush or paper towel to wipe away any dirt.

PER SERVING Calories: 336; Total Fat: 27g; Total Carbs: 7g; Sugar: 5g; Fiber: 1g; Protein: 18g; Sodium: 656mg

THE EASY ANTI-INFLAMMATORY DIET

Smoked Salmon Scrambled Eggs

SERVES 4 / PREP TIME 5 MINUTES / COOK TIME 8 MINUTES

Smoked salmon is salty, so this recipe doesn't contain added salt. If you don't want to use smoked salmon, use fresh cooked or canned salmon and add ½ teaspoon sea salt to the eggs.

2 TABLESPOONS EXTRA-VIRGIN OLIVE OIL

6 OUNCES SMOKED SALMON, FLAKED

8 EGGS, BEATEN

¼ TEASPOON FRESHLY GROUND BLACK PEPPER

1. In a large nonstick skillet over medium-high heat, heat the olive oil until it shimmers.

2. Add the salmon and cook for 3 minutes, stirring.

3. In a medium bowl, whisk the eggs and pepper. Add them to the skillet and cook for about 5 minutes, stirring gently, until done.

PER SERVING Calories: 236; Total Fat: 18g; Total Carbs: <1g; Sugar: <1g; Fiber: 0g; Protein: 19g; Sodium: 974mg

EXTRA-VIRGIN OLIVE OIL

SALMON

DAIRY-FREE
GLUTEN-FREE
NUT-FREE

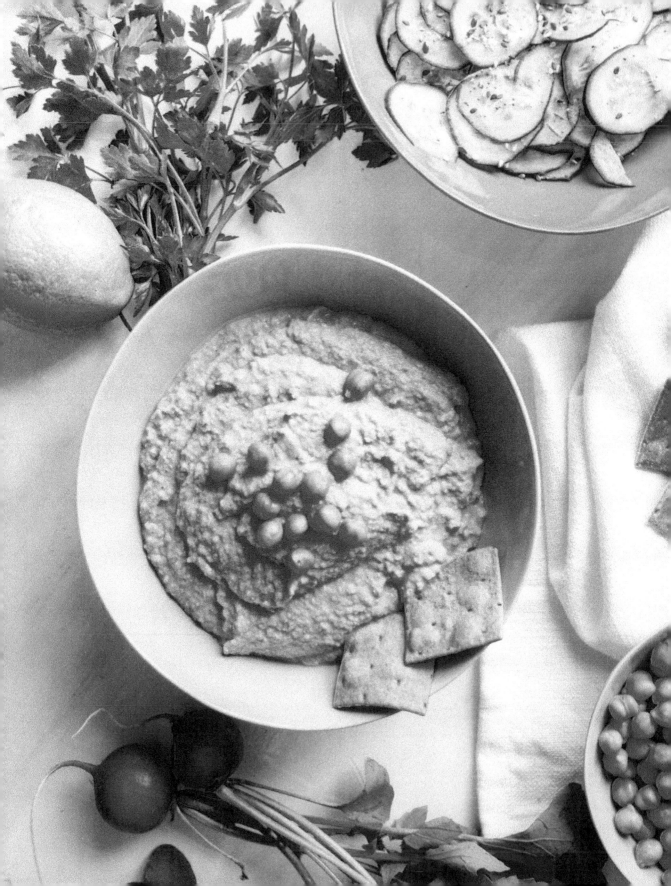

3

SNACKS & SIDES

‹‹ Chickpea and Garlic Hummus, page 42

BROCCOLI

GARLIC

GINGER

DAIRY-FREE
GLUTEN-FREE
NUT-FREE
ONE POT
VEGAN

Broccoli-Sesame Stir-Fry

SERVES 4 / PREP TIME 10 MINUTES / COOK TIME 8 MINUTES

This is one of my favorite ways to enjoy broccoli. It just fits perfectly with the sesame flavor. If you can find it, use expeller-pressed sesame oil instead of toasted sesame oil. While the flavor isn't as strong, it's less processed. If you can't find it, use toasted sesame oil. The overall amount is small and shouldn't contribute to inflammation.

2 TABLESPOONS EXTRA-VIRGIN OLIVE OIL

1 TEASPOON SESAME OIL

4 CUPS BROCCOLI FLORETS

1 TABLESPOON GRATED FRESH GINGER

¼ TEASPOON SEA SALT

2 GARLIC CLOVES, MINCED

2 TABLESPOONS TOASTED SESAME SEEDS

1. In a large nonstick skillet over medium-high heat, heat the olive oil and sesame oil until they shimmer.

2. Add the broccoli, ginger, and salt. Cook for 5 to 7 minutes, stirring frequently, until the broccoli begins to brown.

3. Add the garlic. Cook for 30 seconds, stirring constantly.

4. Remove from the heat and stir in the sesame seeds.

INGREDIENT TIP: Most salad bars have broccoli florets, and you can find bags of broccoli florets in the produce section as well. To save time, buy precut florets.

PER SERVING Calories: 134; Total Fat: 11g; Total Carbs: 9g; Sugar: 2g; Fiber: 3g; Protein: 4g; Sodium: 148mg

Salmon and Dill Pâté

SERVES 4 / PREP TIME 10 MINUTES

SALMON

GLUTEN-FREE
NUT-FREE
ONE POT

Use this as a dip for veggies (red bell pepper slices are great), spread it on celery, or top your favorite nut-based crackers. Purchasing precooked salmon (available in cans and bags near the canned tuna) makes this recipe ready in one simple step.

6 OUNCES COOKED SALMON, BONES AND SKIN REMOVED

¼ CUP HEAVY (WHIPPING) CREAM

1 TABLESPOON CHOPPED FRESH DILL OR 1½ TEASPOONS DRIED

ZEST OF 1 LEMON

½ TEASPOON SEA SALT

In a blender or food processor (or in a large bowl using a mixer), combine the salmon, heavy cream, dill, lemon zest, and salt. Blend until smooth.

SUBSTITUTION TIP: To make this dairy free, replace the heavy cream with ¼ cup full-fat coconut milk.

PER SERVING Calories: 197; Total Fat: 11g; Total Carbs: <1g; Sugar: 0g; Fiber: <1g; Protein: 25g; Sodium: 295mg

EXTRA-VIRGIN
OLIVE OIL

GARLIC

DAIRY-FREE
GLUTEN-FREE
NUT-FREE
ONE POT
VEGAN

Chickpea and Garlic Hummus

SERVES 6 / PREP TIME 5 MINUTES

Hummus is a super-easy snack. Just toss the ingredients in a blender or food processor and process until smooth, garnishing with a shake of paprika and/or some extra-virgin olive oil. Use flatbread or veggies to dip in the hummus for a tasty snack.

3 GARLIC CLOVES, MINCED

2 TABLESPOONS EXTRA-VIRGIN OLIVE OIL (PLUS EXTRA FOR GARNISH, IF DESIRED)

2 TABLESPOONS TAHINI

1 (14-OUNCE) CAN CHICKPEAS, DRAINED

JUICE OF 1 LEMON

½ TEASPOON SEA SALT

PAPRIKA, FOR GARNISH (OPTIONAL)

In a blender or food processor, combine the garlic, olive oil, tahini, chickpeas, lemon juice, and salt. Blend until smooth. Garnish as desired.

PER SERVING Calories: 178; Total Fat: 9g; Total Carbs: 19g; Sugar: 3g; Fiber: 6g; Protein: 7g; Sodium: 171mg

Sautéed Apples and Ginger

SERVES 4 / PREP TIME 10 MINUTES / COOK TIME 10 MINUTES

This complementary side dish for pork or beef also makes a light snack or dessert and brightens plain yogurt for breakfast. In other words, this is one versatile recipe that will fill your kitchen with fabulous fragrance.

2 TABLESPOONS COCONUT OIL	1 TEASPOON GROUND CINNAMON
3 APPLES, PEELED, CORED, AND SLICED	1 PACKET STEVIA
1 TABLESPOON GRATED FRESH GINGER	PINCH SEA SALT

1. In a large nonstick skillet over medium-high heat, heat the coconut oil until it shimmers.

2. Add the apples, ginger, cinnamon, stevia, and salt. Cook for 7 to 10 minutes, stirring occasionally, until the apples are soft.

PER SERVING Calories: 152; Total Fat: 7g; Total Carbs: 24g; Sugar: 18g; Fiber: 5g; Protein: <1g; Sodium: 60mg

CINNAMON

GINGER

DAIRY-FREE
GLUTEN-FREE
ONE POT
VEGAN

**EXTRA-VIRGIN
OLIVE OIL**

GARLIC

SPINACH

DAIRY-FREE
GLUTEN-FREE
NUT-FREE
ONE POT
VEGAN

Citrus Spinach

SERVES 4 / PREP TIME 10 MINUTES / COOK TIME 7 MINUTES

Spinach and orange have a natural affinity for one another. Adding both the orange zest and juice pumps up the citrus flavor. A fantastic side dish for any type of fish or seafood, I like to quickly sauté sea scallops and serve them on a bed of this spinach.

2 TABLESPOONS EXTRA-VIRGIN OLIVE OIL

4 CUPS FRESH BABY SPINACH

2 GARLIC CLOVES, MINCED

JUICE OF ½ ORANGE

ZEST OF ½ ORANGE

½ TEASPOON SEA SALT

⅛ TEASPOON FRESHLY GROUND BLACK PEPPER

1. In a large skillet over medium-high heat, heat the olive oil until it shimmers.

2. Add the spinach and cook for 3 minutes, stirring occasionally.

3. Add the garlic. Cook for 30 seconds, stirring constantly.

4. Add the orange juice, orange zest, salt, and pepper. Cook for about 2 minutes, stirring constantly, until the juice evaporates.

SUBSTITUTION TIP: Try this with Swiss chard or kale. Both are superfood greens that are also beneficial for inflammation with slightly stronger flavors than spinach.

PER SERVING Calories: 80; Total Fat: 7g; Total Carbs: 4g; Sugar: 2g; Fiber: 1g; Protein: 1g; Sodium: 258mg

Rosemary and Garlic Sweet Potatoes

SERVES 4 / PREP TIME 10 MINUTES / COOK TIME 15 MINUTES

I like this as a side dish, but it also makes a fabulous breakfast hash. Just top it with a fried or poached egg for a real treat. I can't get enough of the flavor of rosemary with the caramelization of the sweet potatoes—the garlic just makes them extra-fragrant.

2 TABLESPOONS EXTRA-VIRGIN OLIVE OIL

2 SWEET POTATOES (SKIN LEFT ON), CUT INTO ½-INCH CUBES

1 TABLESPOON CHOPPED FRESH ROSEMARY LEAVES

½ TEASPOON SEA SALT

3 GARLIC CLOVES, MINCED

¼ TEASPOON FRESHLY GROUND BLACK PEPPER

1. In a large nonstick skillet over medium-high heat, heat the olive oil until it shimmers.

2. Add the sweet potatoes, rosemary, and salt. Cook for 10 to 15 minutes, stirring occasionally, until the sweet potatoes begin to brown.

3. Add the garlic and pepper. Cook for 30 seconds, stirring constantly.

PER SERVING Calories: 199; Total Fat: 7g; Total Carbs: 33g; Sugar: <1g; Fiber: 5g; Protein: 2g; Sodium: 245mg

EXTRA-VIRGIN OLIVE OIL

GARLIC

ROSEMARY

DAIRY-FREE
GLUTEN-FREE
NUT-FREE
ONE POT
VEGAN

EXTRA-VIRGIN
OLIVE OIL

RED BELL
PEPPERS

GREEN BELL
PEPPERS

DAIRY-FREE
NUT-FREE
ONE POT
VEGAN

Brown Rice with Bell Peppers

SERVES 4 / PREP TIME 10 MINUTES / COOK TIME 10 MINUTES

The trick to making this dish quick and easy? Buy precooked brown rice, which is available in the grains aisle or freezer section of most grocery stores. With precooked rice, all you need to do is cook the veggies, warm the rice, mix it all together, and it's on the table in about 20 minutes.

2 TABLESPOONS EXTRA-VIRGIN OLIVE OIL

1 RED BELL PEPPER, CHOPPED

1 GREEN BELL PEPPER, CHOPPED

1 ONION, CHOPPED

2 CUPS COOKED BROWN RICE

2 TABLESPOONS LOW-SODIUM SOY SAUCE

1. In a large nonstick skillet over medium-high heat, heat the olive oil until it shimmers.

2. Add the red and green bell peppers and onion. Cook for about 7 minutes, stirring frequently, until the vegetables start to brown.

3. Add the rice and the soy sauce. Cook for about 3 minutes, stirring constantly, until the rice warms through.

INGREDIENT TIP: Save some money by precooking your own brown rice. Do it on a weekend when you have a little extra time. Freeze it in 1-cup portions in resealable bags. It will keep for 3 to 6 months. Just thaw it when you need it.

PER SERVING Calories: 266; Total Fat: 8g; Total Carbs: 44g; Sugar: 4g; Fiber: 3g; Protein: 5g; Sodium: 455mg

THE EASY ANTI-INFLAMMATORY DIET

Garlic Ranch Dip

SERVES 4 / PREP TIME 10 MINUTES

This recipe incorporates the Anti-Inflammatory Mayonnaise (page 148) as well as a little buttermilk. If desired, replace the buttermilk with an equal amount of plain coconut yogurt or almond yogurt and a tablespoon of freshly squeezed lemon juice to make this vegan. Serve it with chopped veggies like red bell peppers and carrots. This also makes a flavorful salad dressing, especially if you thin it with a few tablespoons of water to reach your desired thickness.

¼ CUP ANTI-INFLAMMATORY MAYONNAISE (PAGE 148)

¼ CUP BUTTERMILK

3 GARLIC CLOVES, MINCED

1 TABLESPOON CHOPPED FRESH CHIVES

1 TABLESPOON CHOPPED FRESH DILL

½ TEASPOON SEA SALT

¼ TEASPOON FRESHLY GROUND BLACK PEPPER

In a small bowl, stir together the mayonnaise, buttermilk, garlic, chives, dill, salt, and pepper.

PER SERVING (2 TABLESPOONS) Calories: 69; Total Fat: 5g; Total Carbs: 6g; Sugar: 2g; Fiber: <1g; Protein: 1g; Sodium: 357mg

EXTRA-VIRGIN OLIVE OIL

GARLIC

GLUTEN-FREE
NUT-FREE
ONE POT
VEGETARIAN

GARLIC

DAIRY-FREE
GLUTEN-FREE
NUT-FREE
ONE POT
VEGAN

Guacamole

SERVES 4 / PREP TIME 10 MINUTES

Avocados are a great anti-inflammatory food: They have a beneficial fatty acid profile and are super-creamy to boot. Serve this guacamole with veggies like sliced jicama for dipping, or use it to top fish tacos or some other main dish.

2 AVOCADOS, PEELED, PITTED, AND CUBED

½ RED ONION, MINCED

2 GARLIC CLOVES, FINELY MINCED

JUICE OF 1 LIME

2 TABLESPOONS CHOPPED FRESH CILANTRO LEAVES

½ TEASPOON SEA SALT

In a medium bowl, combine the avocados, red onion, garlic, lime juice, cilantro, and salt. Lightly mash with a fork to mix.

INGREDIENT TIP: To cut an avocado, slice it in half lengthwise (through the poles) and remove the pit. Use a sharp knife to cut cubes into the flesh. Using a big spoon, scoop the flesh from the skin.

PER SERVING Calories: 215; Total Fat: 20g; Total Carbs: 11g; Sugar: 1g; Fiber: 7g; Protein: 2g; Sodium: 243mg

THE EASY ANTI-INFLAMMATORY DIET

Blueberry Nut Trail Mix

SERVES 4 / PREP TIME 5 MINUTES / COOK TIME 5 MINUTES

Dried blueberries still have all the nutritious potency of fresh, and they make a great addition to nuts in this trail mix that has a surprising hit of heat due to Chinese five-spice powder.

1 TABLESPOON EXTRA-VIRGIN OLIVE OIL

1 CUP ALMONDS

PINCH SALT

½ TEASPOON CHINESE FIVE-SPICE POWDER

½ CUP DRIED BLUEBERRIES

1. In a large nonstick skillet over medium-high heat, heat the olive oil until it shimmers.

2. Add the almonds, salt, and Chinese five-spice and cook for 2 minutes, stirring constantly.

3. Remove from the heat and cool. Stir in the blueberries.

PER SERVING Calories: 179; Total Fat: 16g; Total Carbs: 8g; Sugar: 3g; Fiber: 3g; Protein: 5g; Sodium: 39mg

EXTRA-VIRGIN OLIVE OIL

ALMONDS

BLUEBERRIES

DAIRY-FREE
GLUTEN-FREE
ONE POT
VEGAN

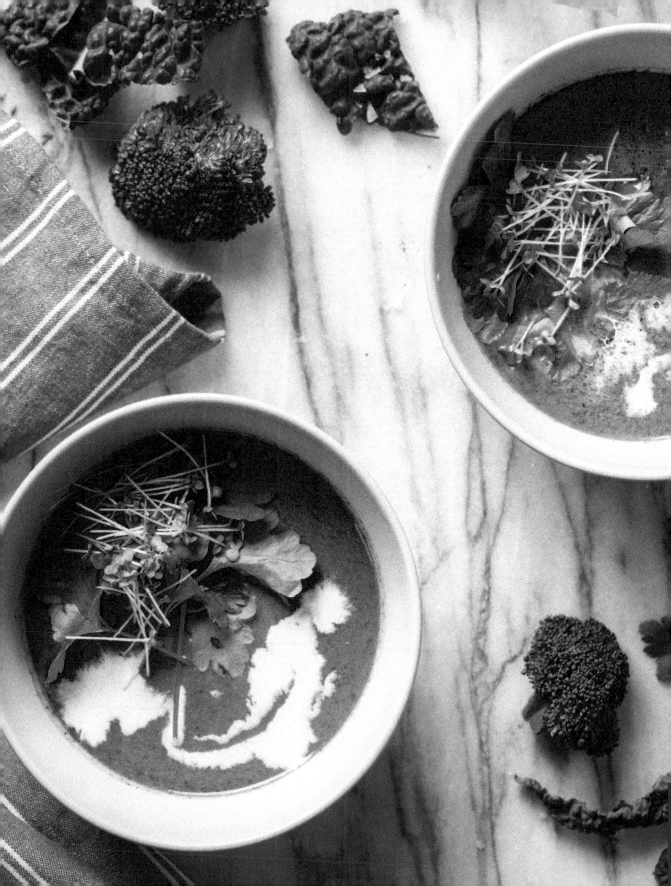

4

SOUPS & SALADS

‹‹ Cream of Kale Soup, page 58

SPINACH

WALNUTS

EXTRA-VIRGIN
OLIVE OIL

DAIRY-FREE
GLUTEN-FREE
VEGAN

Spinach and Walnut Salad with Raspberry Vinaigrette

SERVES 4 / PREP TIME 10 MINUTES

Raspberry vinaigrette has a refreshing acidity that's a lively counter-point to the spinach and rich flavor of walnuts. This is a convenient take-it-with-you salad, but wait to add the vinaigrette until just before serving.

4 CUPS FRESH BABY SPINACH

¼ CUP WALNUT PIECES

¼ CUP RASPBERRY VINAIGRETTE (PAGE 152)

1. In a medium bowl, combine the spinach and walnuts.
2. Toss with the vinaigrette and serve immediately.

SUBSTITUTION TIP: Replace the spinach with kale and replace the walnuts with ¼ cup pomegranate seeds. Toss with the vinaigrette for a super-tasty variation.

PER SERVING Calories: 501; Total Fat: 50g; Total Carbs: 9g; Sugar: 2g; Fiber: 5g; Protein: 11g; Sodium: 96mg

Mixed Berry Salad with Ginger

SERVES 4 / PREP TIME 10 MINUTES

Berry salads make a fabulous snack or side dish, and they're also great with yogurt for breakfast or even as a refreshing dessert. This salad is best in summer when you can buy fresh berries at your local farmers' market, but feel free to enjoy this taste of summer year-round from produce available at the grocery store.

1 CUP FRESH BLUEBERRIES

1 CUP FRESH RASPBERRIES

1 CUP FRESH STRAWBERRIES

1 TABLESPOON GRATED FRESH GINGER

ZEST OF 1 ORANGE

JUICE OF 1 ORANGE

In a medium bowl, stir together the blueberries, raspberries, strawberries, ginger, orange zest, and orange juice to mix well.

STORAGE TIP: Freeze this in freezer containers for 3 months, or refrigerate it, tightly sealed, for 2 to 3 days. This also makes a convenient smoothie base. Toss the frozen salad in the blender with a few cups of your favorite unsweetened milk.

PER SERVING Calories: 75; Total Fat: <1g; Total Carbs: 18g; Sugar: 11g; Fiber: 5g; Protein: 1g; Sodium: 1mg

BLUEBERRIES

GINGER

DAIRY-FREE
GLUTEN-FREE
NUT-FREE
ONE POT
VEGAN

TOMATO

GARLIC

EXTRA-VIRGIN
OLIVE OIL

DAIRY-FREE
GLUTEN-FREE
NUT-FREE
ONE POT
VEGAN

Tomato and Basil Salad

SERVES 4 / PREP TIME 10 MINUTES

This is the quintessential summer salad with tomatoes at their peak of ripeness. I really enjoy my local farmers' market, where I buy heirloom tomatoes, fresh basil, and fresh garlic. If you have that option available, I highly recommend it because the flavor of the final dish will be out of this world.

4 LARGE HEIRLOOM TOMATOES, CHOPPED

¼ CUP FRESH BASIL LEAVES, TORN

2 GARLIC CLOVES, FINELY MINCED

¼ CUP EXTRA-VIRGIN OLIVE OIL

½ TEASPOON SEA SALT

¼ TEASPOON FRESHLY GROUND BLACK PEPPER

In a medium bowl, gently mix together the tomatoes, basil, garlic, olive oil, salt, and pepper.

SUBSTITUTION TIP: If you aren't allergic to or sensitive to dairy, make this into a Caprese salad by adding slices of fresh mozzarella, using about ½ cup altogether. It makes a satisfying meal-size salad.

PER SERVING Calories: 140; Total Fat: 14g; Total Carbs: 4g; Sugar: 3g; Fiber: 1g; Protein: 1g; Sodium: 239mg

Pear-Walnut Salad

SERVES 4 / PREP TIME 10 MINUTES

Pears and walnuts are a classic flavor combination. This recipe makes a nice fruit salad or an irresistible breakfast side dish. Feel free to change the nuts (try hazelnuts in place of the walnuts) or use different types of pears.

4 PEARS, PEELED, CORED, AND CHOPPED

¼ CUP WALNUTS, CHOPPED

2 TABLESPOONS HONEY

2 TABLESPOONS BALSAMIC VINEGAR

2 TABLESPOONS EXTRA-VIRGIN OLIVE OIL

1. In a medium bowl, combine the pears and walnuts.

2. In a small bowl, whisk the honey, balsamic vinegar, and olive oil. Toss with the pears and walnuts.

VARIATION TIP: For a tasty variation, replace the pears with Asian pears. For the vinaigrette, replace the balsamic vinegar with rice vinegar and add 1 tablespoon grated fresh ginger and 1 teaspoon grated orange zest.

PER SERVING Calories: 263; Total Fat: 12g; Total Carbs: 41g; Sugar: 29g; Fiber: 7g; Protein: 3g; Sodium: 3mg

WALNUTS

EXTRA-VIRGIN OLIVE OIL

DAIRY-FREE
GLUTEN-FREE
VEGETARIAN

**EXTRA-VIRGIN
OLIVE OIL**

GARLIC

TOMATOES

DAIRY-FREE
GLUTEN-FREE
NUT-FREE
ONE POT
VEGAN

Tomato Soup

SERVES 4 / PREP TIME 10 MINUTES / COOK TIME 15 MINUTES

This is a simple tomato soup that's tasty by itself as a meal starter or light lunch, or as a sandwich accompaniment. It uses canned tomatoes—my favorite brand is Muir Glen, which offers sugar-free tomatoes with a just-picked flavor.

2 TABLESPOONS EXTRA-VIRGIN OLIVE OIL

1 ONION, FINELY CHOPPED

2 GARLIC CLOVES, MINCED

2 (28-OUNCE) CANS CRUSHED TOMATOES, UNDRAINED

4 CUPS NO-SALT-ADDED VEGETABLE BROTH

½ TEASPOON SEA SALT

⅛ TEASPOON FRESHLY GROUND BLACK PEPPER

1. In a large pot over medium-high heat, heat the olive oil until it shimmers.

2. Add the onion. Cook for about 7 minutes, stirring occasionally, until browned.

3. Add the garlic. Cook for 30 seconds, stirring constantly.

4. Stir in the tomatoes, vegetable broth, salt, and pepper. Simmer for 5 minutes.

5. Carefully transfer the soup to a blender or use an immersion blender. Process until smooth. (See Tip for proper handling of hot liquids in a blender.)

PREPARATION TIP: When puréeing hot liquids, it's important to allow steam to escape through the top of the blender and to protect your hand from burning. After you transfer the soup to the blender, let it sit for 30 seconds. Put the lid on and remove the top spout to allow steam to continue to escape. Fold a kitchen towel into quarters and place it over the top of the blender. Place your hand over the towel to hold the lid in place. Blend for 20 seconds; remove the towel to let steam escape. Continue blending in 20-second bursts, about 3 times, with breaks to allow steam to escape, until smooth. Why am I being so insistent about this? My mom once shot hot lentil soup from a blender all over our kitchen ceiling. Fortunately, she didn't burn herself, but scrubbing the ceiling is never fun.

PER SERVING Calories: 233; Total Fat: 7g; Total Carbs: 35g; Sugar: 24g; Fiber: 13g; Protein: 10g; Sodium: 577mg

THE EASY ANTI-INFLAMMATORY DIET

Gingered Chicken and Vegetable Soup

SERVES 4 / PREP TIME 10 MINUTES / COOK TIME 10 MINUTES

The secret to making this soup fast? Rotisserie chicken from the grocery store with the skin removed. You can buy the rotisserie chicken, shred it, and freeze it in 1-cup portions in resealable bags for three to six months, pulling it out as you need it for recipes. It's a great time saver.

2 TABLESPOONS EXTRA-VIRGIN OLIVE OIL

1 ONION, CHOPPED

2 RED BELL PEPPERS, CHOPPED

1 TABLESPOON GRATED FRESH GINGER

3 CUPS SHREDDED ROTISSERIE CHICKEN, SKIN REMOVED

8 CUPS NO-SALT-ADDED CHICKEN BROTH

½ TEASPOON SEA SALT

⅛ TEASPOON FRESHLY GROUND BLACK PEPPER

1. In a large pot over medium-high heat, heat the olive oil until it shimmers.

2. Add the onion, red bell peppers, and ginger. Cook for about 5 minutes, stirring occasionally, until the vegetables are soft.

3. Stir in the chicken, chicken broth, salt, and pepper. Bring to a simmer. Reduce the heat to medium-low and simmer for 5 minutes.

STORAGE TIP: Make big batches of this soup and freeze it in 2-cup portions. It will keep in the freezer for up to 6 months.

PER SERVING Calories: 341; Total Fat: 15g; Total Carbs: 11g; Sugar: 8g; Fiber: 1g; Protein: 40g; Sodium: 577mg

EXTRA-VIRGIN OLIVE OIL

RED BELL PEPPER

GINGER

DAIRY-FREE

GLUTEN-FREE

NUT-FREE

ONE POT

Cream of Kale Soup

SERVES 4 / PREP TIME 10 MINUTES / COOK TIME 20 MINUTES

This vibrant green soup makes a delicious lunch or dinner. The flavor is best when it's freshly made, so make up a batch to eat it on the same day. Feel free to add your own herbs to enhance the flavor.

EXTRA-VIRGIN OLIVE OIL

KALE

BROCCOLI

GARLIC

DAIRY-FREE
GLUTEN-FREE
NUT-FREE
ONE POT
VEGAN

2 TABLESPOONS EXTRA-VIRGIN OLIVE OIL, PLUS EXTRA FOR GARNISH, IF DESIRED

1 ONION, FINELY CHOPPED

4 CUPS KALE

1 CUP BROCCOLI FLORETS

6 CUPS NO-SALT VEGETABLE BROTH

1 TEASPOON GARLIC POWDER

½ TEASPOON SEA SALT

¼ TEASPOON FRESHLY GROUND BLACK PEPPER

MICROGREENS (OPTIONAL)

COCONUT MILK (OPTIONAL)

1. In a large pot over medium-high heat, heat the olive oil until it shimmers.

2. Add the onion and cook about 5 minutes, stirring occasionally, until it is soft.

3. Add the kale, broccoli, vegetable broth, garlic powder, salt, and pepper. Bring to a boil and reduce the heat to medium-low. Simmer 10 to 15 minutes, until the vegetables are soft.

4. Carefully transfer to a blender and blend until smooth. Serve hot with the additional oil, microgreens, and coconut milk, if using.

PER SERVING Calories: 129; Total Fat: 7g; Total Carbs: 16g; Sugar: 6g; Fiber: 2g; Protein: 3g; Sodium: 302mg

Curried Sweet Potato Soup

SERVES 4 / PREP TIME 10 MINUTES / COOK TIME 15 MINUTES

Turmeric is one of the flavors in curry powder and it is especially nice with sweet potatoes. This simple soup has a ton of flavor, making it a satisfying main course you're sure to enjoy.

2 TABLESPOONS EXTRA-VIRGIN OLIVE OIL

1 ONION, CHOPPED

4 CUPS CUBED, PEELED SWEET POTATO

8 CUPS NO-SALT-ADDED VEGETABLE BROTH

1 TEASPOON CURRY POWDER

1 TEASPOON GROUND TURMERIC

½ TEASPOON SEA SALT

⅛ TEASPOON FRESHLY GROUND BLACK PEPPER

1. In a large pot over medium-high heat, heat the olive oil until it shimmers.

2. Add the onion. Cook for about 5 minutes, stirring occasionally, until soft.

3. Stir in the sweet potato, vegetable broth, curry powder, turmeric, salt, and pepper. Bring to a boil. Reduce the heat to medium and simmer for about 10 minutes until the sweet potato cubes are soft.

4. Carefully transfer to a blender and blend until smooth.

PER SERVING Calories: 253; Total Fat: 7g; Total Carbs: 45g; Sugar: 2g; Fiber: 7g; Protein: 3g; Sodium: 261mg

EXTRA-VIRGIN OLIVE OIL

TURMERIC

DAIRY-FREE
GLUTEN-FREE
NUT-FREE
ONE POT
VEGAN

EXTRA-VIRGIN
OLIVE OIL

GINGER

GARLIC

DAIRY-FREE
GLUTEN-FREE
NUT-FREE
ONE POT
VEGAN

Squash and Ginger Soup

SERVES 4 / PREP TIME 10 MINUTES / COOK TIME 20 MINUTES

This quick and easy soup has lots of flavor. Fragrant with anti-inflammatory ginger and garlic, it makes a great main dish or is perfect for making ahead and taking as meals on the go. It will keep in the fridge for three to five days or in the freezer for up to six months.

2 TABLESPOONS EXTRA-VIRGIN
OLIVE OIL

1 ONION, CHOPPED

1 TABLESPOON GRATED GINGER

4 GARLIC CLOVES, MINCED

6 CUPS VEGETABLE BROTH

3 CUPS BUTTERNUT SQUASH
(OR ACORN SQUASH)

½ TEASPOON SEA SALT

¼ TEASPOON FRESHLY GROUND
BLACK PEPPER

¼ CUP COCONUT MILK (OPTIONAL)

¼ CUP MICROGREENS (OPTIONAL)

1. In a large pot over medium-high heat, heat the olive oil until it shimmers.

2. Add the onion and ginger, and cook about 5 minutes, stirring occasionally, until onion is soft.

3. Add the garlic and cook for 30 seconds more, stirring constantly.

4. Add the vegetable broth, squash, salt, and pepper. Cook, covered, for about 10 minutes, until the squash is soft.

5. Carefully transfer to a blender. Blend and blend until smooth.

6. Serve garnished with the coconut milk and microgreens, if using.

SUBSTITUTION TIP: Save time by buying prechopped squash, which is usually available in the produce section of your grocery store, or frozen squash, which is available in the freezer section.

PER SERVING Calories: 96; Total Fat: 7g; Total Carbs: 9g; Sugar: 6g; Fiber: <1g; Protein: <1g; Sodium 266mg

GREEN TEA

GLUTEN-FREE
NUT-FREE
ONE POT
VEGAN

Melon and Green Tea Soup

SERVES 4 / PREP TIME 5 MINUTES

This sweet soup makes a delicious meal starter or dessert. Keep the honeydew in the fridge along with all the other ingredients so the soup is cold.

2 TABLESPOONS MATCHA

2 CUPS CUBED HONEYDEW MELON

2 TABLESPOONS CHOPPED FRESH MINT, PLUS MORE FOR GARNISH

2 TABLESPOONS HONEY

½ CUP WATER

½ CUP NON-FAT GREEK YOGURT

In a blender or food processor, combine the matcha, melon, mint, honey, water, and yogurt. Blend until smooth. Garnish with mint sprigs.

COOKING TIP: If you have some extra time, chill this soup for 30 minutes in the freezer or 1 hour in the fridge so it's extra cold when you serve it.

PER SERVING Calories: 168; Total Fat: <1g; Total Carbs: 40g; Sugar: 36g; Fiber: 3g; Protein: 5g; Sodium: 73mg

Easy Summer Gazpacho

SERVES 4 / PREP TIME 10 MINUTES

It wasn't until I was an adult that I came to truly appreciate how refreshing cold soup can be— possibly due to a traumatic experience as a child with tomato aspic, which I thought was strawberry gelatin! As a grown-up who has gotten over that experience (mostly), I've come to appreciate the ease of making gazpacho and its fresh and revitalizing flavors convinced me. If, like me, you once were trauma- tized by gelled tomato, head to the farmers' market, get some fresh produce, and give this a try.

TOMATOES

EXTRA-VIRGIN OLIVE OIL

GARLIC

6 LARGE HEIRLOOM TOMATOES, CHOPPED

¼ CUP EXTRA-VIRGIN OLIVE OIL

¼ CUP FRESH BASIL LEAVES

2 GARLIC CLOVES, MINCED

JUICE OF 1 LEMON

ZEST OF 1 LEMON

½ TO 1 TEASPOON HOT SAUCE (OPTIONAL)

DAIRY-FREE
GLUTEN-FREE
NUT-FREE
ONE POT
VEGAN

In a blender, combine the tomatoes, olive oil, basil, garlic, lemon juice and zest, and hot sauce (if using). Pulse 20 times, in 1-second bursts, for a chunkier soup, or continue blending until smooth for a smoother texture.

INGREDIENT TIP: I have a confession to make. I don't mince my garlic. Instead, I use a garlic press, which saves tons of time. Just pop a clove in, squeeze the handle, and out comes perfectly minced garlic.

PER SERVING Calories: 165; Total Fat: 13g; Total Carbs: 12g; Sugar: 8g; Fiber: 3g; Protein: 3g; Sodium: 283mg

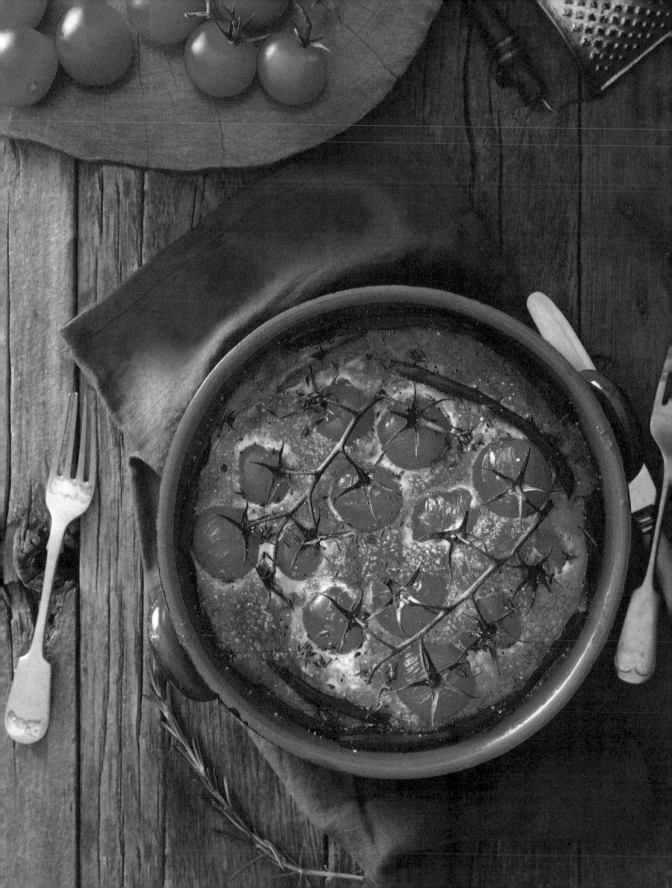

5

VEGETARIAN & VEGAN
DISHES

‹‹ Tomato Asparagus Frittata, page 76

EXTRA-VIRGIN
OLIVE OIL

TURMERIC

TOMATOES

DAIRY-FREE
GLUTEN-FREE
NUT-FREE
ONE POT
VEGAN

Lentils with Tomatoes and Turmeric

SERVES 4 / PREP TIME 10 MINUTES / COOK TIME 10 MINUTES

This delicious lentil stew makes a great vegetarian main when served with brown rice or a scrumptious side dish. Using canned lentils allows them to cook quickly so you'll have dinner on the table in less than 30 minutes.

2 TABLESPOONS EXTRA-VIRGIN OLIVE OIL, PLUS EXTRA FOR GARNISH

1 ONION, FINELY CHOPPED

1 TABLESPOON GROUND TURMERIC

1 TEASPOON GARLIC POWDER

1 (14-OUNCE) CAN LENTILS, DRAINED

1 (14-OUNCE) CAN CHOPPED TOMATOES, DRAINED

½ TEASPOON SEA SALT

¼ TEASPOON FRESHLY GROUND BLACK PEPPER

1. In a large pot over medium-high heat, heat the olive oil until it shimmers.

2. Add the onion and turmeric, and cook for about 5 minutes, stirring occasionally, until soft.

3. Add the garlic powder, lentils, tomatoes, salt, and pepper. Cook for 5 minutes, stirring occasionally. Serve garnished with additional olive oil, if desired

PER SERVING Calories: 248; Total Fat: 8g; Total Carbs: 34g; Sugar: 5g; Fiber: 15g; Protein: 12g; Sodium 243mg

Whole-Wheat Pasta with Tomato-Basil Sauce

SERVES 4 / PREP TIME 15 MINUTES / COOK TIME 10 MINUTES

Whole-wheat pasta isn't gluten free, but there are other gluten-free options available. One of my favorites is turning zucchini into "noodles" using a spiralizer. If you do this, sauté the noodles in olive oil for about five minutes. Otherwise, if you need gluten-free pasta, you can now find some excellent choices at most grocery stores.

2 TABLESPOONS EXTRA-VIRGIN OLIVE OIL

1 ONION, MINCED

6 GARLIC CLOVES, MINCED

2 (28-OUNCE) CANS CRUSHED TOMATOES, UNDRAINED

½ TEASPOON SEA SALT

¼ TEASPOON FRESHLY GROUND BLACK PEPPER

¼ CUP BASIL LEAVES, CHOPPED

1 (8-OUNCE) PACKAGE WHOLE-WHEAT PASTA

1. In a large pot over medium-high heat, heat the olive oil until it shimmers.

2. Add the onion. Cook for about 5 minutes, stirring occasionally, until soft.

3. Add the garlic. Cook for 30 seconds, stirring constantly.

4. Stir in the tomatoes, salt, and pepper. Bring to a simmer. Reduce the heat to medium and cook for 5 minutes, stirring occasionally.

5. Remove from the heat and stir in the basil. Toss with the pasta.

INGREDIENT TIP: For even more flavor, buy canned tomatoes that have basil and garlic in them. Don't change the rest of the recipe though, this just pumps up the flavor even more.

PER SERVING Calories: 330; Total Fat: 8g; Total Carbs: 56g; Sugar: 24g; Fiber: 17g; Protein: 14g; Sodium: 1,000mg

EXTRA-VIRGIN OLIVE OIL

GARLIC

TOMATOES

DAIRY-FREE

NUT-FREE

VEGAN

EXTRA-VIRGIN
OLIVE OIL

KALE

GARLIC

GINGER

DAIRY-FREE
NUT-FREE
ONE POT
VEGAN

Fried Rice with Kale

SERVES 4 / PREP TIME 10 MINUTES / COOK TIME 12 MINUTES

Using pre-cooked rice saves time when making this recipe. Tofu adds a little protein, and the Stir-Fry Sauce (page 149) adds lots of flavor. To make this gluten free, use tamari or gluten-free soy sauce.

2 TABLESPOONS EXTRA-VIRGIN OLIVE OIL

8 OUNCES TOFU, CHOPPED

6 SCALLIONS, WHITE AND GREEN PARTS, THINLY SLICED

2 CUPS KALE, STEMMED AND CHOPPED

3 CUPS COOKED BROWN RICE

¼ CUP STIR-FRY SAUCE (PAGE 149)

1. In a large skillet over medium-high heat, heat the olive oil until it shimmers.

2. Add the tofu, scallions, and kale. Cook for 5 to 7 minutes, stirring frequently, until the vegetables are soft.

3. Add the brown rice and stir-fry sauce. Cook for 3 to 5 minutes, stirring occasionally, until heated through.

STORAGE TIP: This freezes well. Store 1-cup portions in tightly sealed containers in the freezer for up to 6 months.

PER SERVING Calories: 301; Total Fat: 11g; Total Carbs: 36g; Sugar: 1g; Fiber: 3g; Protein: 16g; Sodium: 2,535mg

Tofu and Spinach Sauté

SERVES 4 / PREP TIME 10 MINUTES / COOK TIME 10 MINUTES

Tofu is an excellent source of vegetable protein if you're not sensitive to soy. You can use any type of tofu here. I like the extra-firm silken tofu, which has a lower moisture content than other types, but any extra-firm or firm variety will offer robust texture.

2 TABLESPOONS EXTRA-VIRGIN OLIVE OIL

1 ONION, CHOPPED

4 CUPS FRESH BABY SPINACH

8 OUNCES TOFU

3 GARLIC CLOVES, MINCED

JUICE OF 1 ORANGE

ZEST OF 1 ORANGE

½ TEASPOON SEA SALT

⅛ TEASPOON FRESHLY GROUND BLACK PEPPER

1. In a large skillet over medium-high heat, heat the olive oil until it shimmers.

2. Add the onion, spinach, and tofu. Cook for about 5 minutes, stirring occasionally, until the onion is soft.

3. Add the garlic. Cook for 30 seconds, stirring constantly.

4. Add the orange juice, orange zest, salt, and pepper. Cook for 3 minutes, stirring, until heated through.

INGREDIENT TIP: If you buy regular tofu (not extra-firm silken tofu), you can remove some water content by slicing it and placing it in a colander. Put the colander in a sink with a plate on top and something weighting the plate (canned goods work well). Let it sit for about 30 minutes, and the tofu will firm up as the water drains.

PER SERVING Calories: 128; Total Fat: 10g; Total Carbs: 7g; Sugar: 3g; Fiber: 2g; Protein: 6g; Sodium: 266mg

EXTRA-VIRGIN OLIVE OIL

SPINACH

GARLIC

DAIRY-FREE
GLUTEN-FREE
NUT-FREE
ONE POT
VEGAN

EXTRA-VIRGIN OLIVE OIL

RED BELL PEPPER

GINGER

GARLIC

DAIRY-FREE
NUT-FREE
ONE POT
VEGAN

Tofu and Red Pepper Stir-Fry

SERVES 4 / PREP TIME 10 MINUTES / COOK TIME 11 MINUTES

If you need this dish to be gluten free, replace the soy sauce with gluten-free soy sauce, tamari (which is naturally gluten free), or even coconut aminos. You'll still get the umami flavor of the soy sauce without the wheat and gluten.

2 TABLESPOONS EXTRA-VIRGIN OLIVE OIL

2 RED BELL PEPPERS, CHOPPED

1 ONION, CHOPPED

8 OUNCES TOFU, CHOPPED

1 RECIPE GINGER-TERIYAKI SAUCE (PAGE 150)

1. In a large skillet over medium-high heat, heat the olive oil until it shimmers.

2. Add the red bell peppers, onion, and tofu. Cook for 5 to 7 minutes, stirring occasionally, until the vegetables are soft and begin to brown.

3. Whisk the teriyaki sauce and add it to the skillet. Cook for 3 to 4 minutes, stirring, until the sauce thickens.

PER SERVING Calories: 166; Total Fat: 10g; Total Carbs: 17g; Sugar: 12g; Fiber: 2g; Protein: 7g; Sodium: 892mg

Sweet Potato Curry with Spinach

SERVES 4 / PREP TIME 10 MINUTES / COOK TIME 20 MINUTES

Curry is one of my favorite meals—it's so warming, and sweet potatoes are perfect for a slightly spicy curry. It takes 15 to 20 minutes to cook potatoes to tender, but they are filled with flavor from simmering in the fragrant liquid in this one-pot meal. While this recipe has a few extra ingredients, they are pantry staples you'll have on hand if you followed the pantry essentials list on page 20.

EXTRA-VIRGIN OLIVE OIL

SPINACH

DAIRY-FREE
GLUTEN-FREE
ONE POT
VEGAN

2 TABLESPOONS EXTRA-VIRGIN OLIVE OIL

1 ONION, CHOPPED

4 CUPS CUBED PEELED SWEET POTATO

4 CUPS FRESH BABY SPINACH

3 CUPS NO-SALT-ADDED VEGETABLE BROTH

1 CUP LITE COCONUT MILK

2 TABLESPOONS CURRY POWDER

½ TEASPOON SEA SALT

⅛ TEASPOON FRESHLY GROUND BLACK PEPPER

1. In a large pot over medium-high heat, heat the olive oil until it shimmers.

2. Add the onion. Cook for about 5 minutes, stirring, until soft.

3. Stir in the sweet potato, spinach, vegetable broth, coconut milk, curry powder, salt, and pepper. Bring to a simmer and reduce the heat to medium. Cook for about 15 minutes, stirring occasionally, until the sweet potatoes are soft.

INGREDIENT TIP: Here's a fun idea for sweet potatoes that helps them cook more quickly and gives you more of a "pasta" experience. Using a vegetable peeler, peel the sweet potatoes into strips and then cut the strips into long, flat noodles. This will reduce the cooking time by about half. I've also found sweet potatoes pre-cut this way in bags with the prepped veggies at my local grocery store.

PER SERVING Calories: 314; Total Fat: 11g; Total Carbs: 50g; Sugar: 14g; Fiber: 9g; Protein: 8g; Sodium: 400mg

EXTRA-VIRGIN
OLIVE OIL

RED BELL
PEPPER

DAIRY-FREE
GLUTEN-FREE
NUT-FREE
ONE POT
VEGETARIAN

Sweet Potato and Bell Pepper Hash with a Fried Egg

SERVES 4 / PREP TIME 5 MINUTES / COOK TIME 25 MINUTES

While many people think of eggs and hash as a breakfast staple, I really enjoy this dish for dinner. I find it hearty, satisfying, and totally delicious, and the sweet potatoes and sweetness of the bell peppers complement each other well.

4 TABLESPOONS EXTRA-VIRGIN OLIVE OIL, DIVIDED

1 ONION, CHOPPED

1 RED BELL PEPPER, CHOPPED

4 CUPS CUBED, PEELED SWEET POTATO

1 TEASPOON SEA SALT, DIVIDED

⅛ TEASPOON FRESHLY GROUND BLACK PEPPER

4 EGGS

1. In a large nonstick skillet over medium-high heat, heat 2 tablespoons of the olive oil until it shimmers.

2. Add the onion, red bell pepper, and sweet potato. Season with ½ teaspoon of the salt and the pepper. Cook for 15 to 20 minutes, stirring occasionally, until the sweet potatoes are soft and browned. Divide the potatoes among 4 plates.

3. Return the skillet to the heat, reduce the heat to medium-low, and heat the remaining 2 tablespoons of olive oil, swirling to coat the bottom of the pan.

4. Carefully crack the eggs into the pan and sprinkle with the remaining ½ teaspoon of salt. Cook for 3 to 4 minutes until the whites are set. Gently flip the eggs and turn off the heat. Let the eggs sit in the hot pan for 1 minute. Place 1 egg on top of each serving of hash.

PER SERVING Calories: 384; Total Fat: 19g; Total Carbs: 47g; Sugar: 16g; Fiber: 8g; Protein: 10g; Sodium: 603mg

THE EASY ANTI-INFLAMMATORY DIET

Buckwheat Noodles with Peanut Sauce

SERVES 4 / PREP TIME 20 MINUTES

Many people are surprised to learn that buckwheat is gluten free. It's not wheat or a grain, but rather a seed. If gluten is an issue for you, read the package label carefully to ensure that it contains no wheat. The label should list only buckwheat flour and no wheat of any kind.

1 (8-OUNCE) PACKAGE BUCKWHEAT NOODLES, COOKED ACCORDING TO PACKAGE DIRECTIONS AND DRAINED

1 RECIPE PEANUT SAUCE (PAGE 154)

¼ CUP FRESH CILANTRO LEAVES, CHOPPED

¼ CUP PEANUTS, CHOPPED

6 SCALLIONS, WHITE AND GREEN PARTS, THINLY SLICED DIAGONALLY

In a large bowl, toss the buckwheat noodles with the peanut sauce to coat. Garnish with the cilantro, peanuts, and scallions.

SUBSTITUTION TIP: If you're allergic to peanuts, replace the peanut butter (in the sauce) and peanuts with almond or cashew butter and chopped almonds or cashews.

PER SERVING Calories: 388; Total Fat: 18g; Total Carbs: 51g; Sugar: 4g; Fiber: 8g; Protein: 16g; Sodium: 542mg

PEANUTS

GINGER

DAIRY-FREE
GLUTEN-FREE
VEGAN

**EXTRA-VIRGIN
OLIVE OIL**

SPINACH

GARLIC

DAIRY-FREE
GLUTEN-FREE
NUT-FREE
ONE POT
VEGAN

Quinoa Florentine

SERVES 4 / PREP TIME 5 MINUTES / COOK TIME 25 MINUTES

Florentine is the culinary way of saying "with spinach." You can use any type of quinoa (pronounced KEEN-wah) here. I'm partial to red quinoa, but that's a bit harder to locate, so use whatever type you can find for this warming and satisfying dish.

2 TABLESPOONS EXTRA-VIRGIN
OLIVE OIL

1 ONION, CHOPPED

3 CUPS FRESH BABY SPINACH

3 GARLIC CLOVES, MINCED

2 CUPS QUINOA, RINSED WELL

4 CUPS NO-SALT-ADDED
VEGETABLE BROTH

½ TEASPOON SEA SALT

⅛ TEASPOON FRESHLY GROUND
BLACK PEPPER

1. In a large pot over medium-high heat, heat the olive oil until it shimmers.

2. Add the onion and spinach. Cook for 3 minutes, stirring occasionally.

3. Add the garlic and cook for 30 seconds, stirring constantly.

4. Stir in the quinoa, vegetable broth, salt, and pepper. Bring to a boil and reduce the heat to low. Cover and simmer for 15 to 20 minutes, until the liquid is absorbed. Fluff with a fork.

PER SERVING Calories: 403; Total Fat: 12g; Total Carbs: 62g; Sugar: 4g; Fiber: 7g; Protein: 13g; Sodium: 278mg

Kale Frittata

SERVES 4 / PREP TIME 10 MINUTES / COOK TIME 17 MINUTES

Greens and eggs make a colorful and nutritious meal. While many people consider frittatas breakfast food, I like them for lunch or dinner. They transport and reheat well, so they're especially good to take for lunches on the go. Simply microwave a wedge for 60 to 90 seconds depending on your microwave's power.

2 TABLESPOONS EXTRA-VIRGIN OLIVE OIL

4 CUPS STEMMED AND CHOPPED KALE

3 GARLIC CLOVES, MINCED

8 EGGS

½ TEASPOON SEA SALT

¼ TEASPOON FRESHLY GROUND BLACK PEPPER

2 TABLESPOONS SUNFLOWER SEEDS

1. Preheat the broiler to high.

2. In a large ovenproof skillet over medium-high heat, heat the olive oil until it shimmers.

3. Add the kale. Cook for about 5 minutes, stirring, until soft.

4. Add the garlic. Cook for 30 seconds, stirring constantly.

5. In a medium bowl, beat the eggs, salt, and pepper. Carefully pour them over the kale. Reduce the heat to medium. Cook the eggs for about 3 minutes until set around the edges. Using a rubber spatula, carefully pull the eggs away from the edges of the skillet and tilt the pan to let the uncooked eggs run into the edges. Cook for about 3 minutes, until the edges set again.

6. Sprinkle with the sunflower seeds. Transfer the pan to the broiler and cook for 3 to 5 minutes until puffed and brown. Cut into wedges to serve.

PREPARATION TIP: Boost the anti-inflammatory power and add more color and flavor. Chop an heirloom tomato and sprinkle it over the frittata before serving.

PER SERVING Calories: 231; Total Fat: 17g; Total Carbs: 9g; Sugar: <1g; Fiber: 1g; Protein: 14g; Sodium: 387mg

EXTRA-VIRGIN OLIVE OIL

KALE

GARLIC

DAIRY-FREE
GLUTEN-FREE
NUT-FREE
VEGETARIAN

**EXTRA-VIRGIN
OLIVE OIL**

TOMATO

DAIRY-FREE
GLUTEN-FREE
NUT-FREE
VEGETARIAN

Tomato Asparagus Frittata

SERVES 4 / PREP TIME 10 MINUTES / COOK TIME 10 MINUTES

Frittatas make a fabulous meal at any time of day because they are quick, easy, and can be varied endlessly for your own flavor preferences. They also keep well—slice them into single serving wedges and freeze them in resealable bags in individual servings for up to 6 months.

2 TABLESPOONS EXTRA-VIRGIN OLIVE OIL

10 ASPARAGUS SPEARS, TRIMMED

10 CHERRY TOMATOES

6 EGGS

1 TABLESPOON CHOPPED, FRESH THYME

½ TEASPOON SEA SALT

⅛ TEASPOON FRESHLY GROUND BLACK PEPPER

1. Preheat the broiler to high.

2. In a large ovenproof skillet over medium-high heat, heat the olive oil until it shimmers.

3. Add the asparagus. Cook for 5 minutes, stirring occasionally.

4. Add the tomatoes. Cook 3 minutes, stirring occasionally.

5. In a medium bowl, whisk together the eggs, thyme, salt, and pepper. Carefully pour over the asparagus and tomatoes, moving the vegetables around so they are evenly spread in the pan.

6. Reduce the heat to medium. Cook the eggs for about 3 minutes until set around the edges. Using a rubber spatula, carefully pull the eggs away from the edges of the skillet and tilt the pan to let the uncooked eggs run into the edges. Cook for about 3 minutes, until the edges set again.

7. Carefully transfer the pan to the broiler and cook for 3 to 5 minutes until puffed and brown. Cut into wedges to serve.

PER SERVING Calories: 224; Total Fat: 14g; Total Carbs: 15g; Sugar: 10g; Fiber: 5g; Protein: 12g; Sodium: 343mg

Black Bean Chili with Garlic and Tomatoes

SERVES 4 / PREP TIME 10 MINUTES / COOK TIME 20 MINUTES

Chili is such a versatile dish. Add your favorite flavors and spices, changing the types of beans you use, or adding extra chopped veggies like green or red bell peppers, jalapeños, or carrots. You can even change the heat level by adding cayenne. So go nuts— make this chili your own. (Hint: I like to add a bit of unsweetened cocoa powder to make the flavors richer.)

2 TABLESPOONS EXTRA-VIRGIN OLIVE OIL

1 ONION, CHOPPED

2 (28-OUNCE) CANS CHOPPED TOMATOES, UNDRAINED

2 (14-OUNCE) CANS BLACK BEANS, DRAINED

1 TABLESPOON CHILI POWDER

1 TEASPOON GARLIC POWDER

½ TEASPOON SEA SALT

1. In a large pot over medium-high, heat the olive oil until it shimmers.

2. Add the onion. Cook for about 5 minutes, stirring occasionally, until soft.

3. Stir in the tomatoes, black beans, chili powder, garlic powder, and salt. Bring to a simmer. Reduce the heat to medium and cook for 15 minutes, stirring occasionally.

PREPARATION TIP: This is a perfect recipe for the slow cooker! Toss all the ingredients (raw) into your slow cooker in the morning, set it on low heat, and come back 8 hours later for a flavorful and filling meal.

PER SERVING Calories: 481; Total Fat: 10g; Total Carbs: 80g; Sugar: 14g; Fiber: 21g; Protein: 25g; Sodium: 278mg

EXTRA-VIRGIN OLIVE OIL

TOMATOES

GARLIC

DAIRY-FREE
GLUTEN-FREE
NUT-FREE
ONE POT
VEGAN

**EXTRA-VIRGIN
OLIVE OIL**

TOMATOES

GARLIC

DAIRY-FREE
GLUTEN-FREE
NUT-FREE
ONE POT
VEGAN

Tofu Sloppy Joes

SERVES 4 / PREP TIME 10 MINUTES / COOK TIME 15 MINUTES

I like to eat sloppy Joes in lettuce cups, but you can also put them on buns, use them to top brown rice, or just eat the mixture like a stew. It's up to you! It makes a fun meal that keeps well in the freezer for up to six months.

2 TABLESPOONS EXTRA-VIRGIN OLIVE OIL

1 ONION, CHOPPED

10 OUNCES TOFU, CHOPPED

2 (14-OUNCE) CANS CRUSHED TOMATOES, 1 DRAINED AND 1 UNDRAINED

¼ CUP APPLE CIDER VINEGAR

1 TABLESPOON CHILI POWDER

1 TEASPOON GARLIC POWDER

½ TEASPOON SEA SALT

⅛ TEASPOON FRESHLY GROUND BLACK PEPPER

1. In a large pot over medium-high heat, heat the olive oil until it shimmers.

2. Add the onion and tofu. Cook for about 5 minutes, stirring occasionally, until the onion is soft.

3. Stir in the tomatoes, cider vinegar, chili powder, garlic powder, salt, and pepper. Simmer for 10 minutes to let the flavors blend, stirring occasionally.

PER SERVING Calories: 209; Total Fat: 10g; Total Carbs: 21g; Sugar: 13g; Fiber: 8g; Protein: 11g; Sodium: 644mg

THE EASY ANTI-INFLAMMATORY DIET

Mushroom Pesto Burgers

SERVES 4 / PREP TIME 5 MINUTES / COOK TIME 20 MINUTES

Giant portobello mushroom caps make a hearty and savory meat replacement for burger night. Adding pesto "beefs" up the flavor. You can use whole-wheat or gluten-free buns or eat the mushroom caps sans buns.

4 PORTOBELLO MUSHROOM CAPS, STEMMED, GILLS REMOVED

1 RECIPE SPINACH PESTO (PAGE 147)

4 ONION SLICES

4 TOMATO SLICES

4 WHOLE-WHEAT HAMBURGER BUNS

1. Preheat the oven to 400°F.

2. Brush the mushroom caps on both sides with the pesto to coat and place them on a rimmed baking sheet. Bake for 15 to 20 minutes until soft.

3. Layer the mushrooms on the buns with the tomatoes and onions.

SUBSTITUTION TIP: To make this vegan and dairy free, omit the Parmesan cheese in the pesto or replace it with 2 tablespoons nutritional yeast.

PER SERVING Calories: 339; Total Fat: 23; Total Carbs: 26g; Sugar: 6g; Fiber: 5g; Protein: 12g; Sodium: 278mg

SPINACH

EXTRA-VIRGIN OLIVE OIL

GARLIC

TOMATOES

NUT-FREE

VEGETARIAN

EXTRA-VIRGIN
OLIVE OIL

BROCCOLI

GARLIC

DAIRY-FREE
GLUTEN-FREE
NUT-FREE
VEGETARIAN

Broccoli and Egg "Muffins"

SERVES 4 / PREP TIME 10 MINUTES / COOK TIME 20 MINUTES

Whip up these bite-size eggs for breakfast, lunch, or dinner. They reheat easily in the microwave (60 to 90 seconds), so they are especially suited to meals on the run. They also freeze well and will keep there for three to six months.

NONSTICK COOKING SPRAY

2 TABLESPOONS EXTRA-VIRGIN OLIVE OIL

1 ONION, CHOPPED

1 CUP BROCCOLI FLORETS, CHOPPED

8 EGGS, BEATEN

1 TEASPOON GARLIC POWDER

½ TEASPOON SEA SALT

¼ TEASPOON FRESHLY GROUND BLACK PEPPER

1. Preheat the oven to 350°F.

2. Spray a muffin tin with nonstick cooking spray.

3. In a large nonstick skillet over medium-high heat, heat the olive oil until it shimmers.

4. Add the onion and broccoli. Cook for 3 minutes. Spoon the vegetables evenly into 4 muffin cups.

5. In a medium bowl, beat the eggs, garlic powder, salt, and pepper. Pour them over the vegetables in the muffin cups.

6. Bake for 15 to 17 minutes until the eggs set.

INGREDIENT TIP: This recipe is a good one to use up those broccoli stems if you've used all the florets for another recipe. Simply chop the stems into bite-size pieces.

PER SERVING Calories: 207; Total Fat: 16; Total Carbs: 5g; Sugar: 2g; Fiber: 1g; Protein: 12g; Sodium: 366mg

Egg Salad Cups

SERVES 4 / PREP TIME 10 MINUTES

Here's my secret for perfect hard-boiled eggs. Put them in a single layer in the bottom of a large pot and cover with water by one inch. Put the pot over high heat and bring to a boil. Boil for one minute. Turn off the heat and cover with the lid. Let the eggs sit for 14 minutes. Run them under cold water to stop the cooking. You can also buy peeled, boiled eggs at the grocery store as a time-saver.

8 HARD-BOILED EGGS, PEELED AND CHOPPED

½ RED BELL PEPPER, FINELY CHOPPED

¼ CUP ANTI-INFLAMMATORY MAYONNAISE (PAGE 148)

1 TEASPOON DIJON MUSTARD

½ TEASPOON SEA SALT

⅛ TEASPOON FRESHLY GROUND BLACK PEPPER

4 LARGE LETTUCE LEAVES

1. In a large bowl, combine the eggs, red bell pepper, mayonnaise, mustard, salt, and pepper. Mix gently to combine.

2. Spoon the mixture into the lettuce leaves.

INGREDIENT TIP: Have trouble peeling eggs? Use older eggs, not extremely fresh eggs—they peel better. Gently tap the rounded end of the egg on the counter and run the egg under cold water as you peel it.

PER SERVING Calories: 190; Total Fat: 14; Total Carbs: 6g; Sugar: 2g; Fiber: <1g; Protein: 11g; Sodium: 477mg

EXTRA-VIRGIN OLIVE OIL

RED BELL PEPPER

DAIRY-FREE

GLUTEN-FREE

NUT-FREE

ONE POT

VEGETARIAN

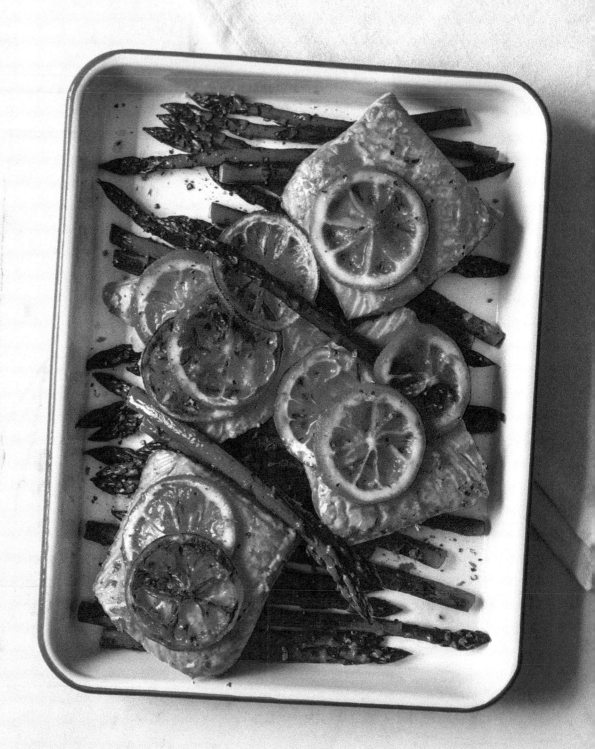

6

SEAFOOD DISHES

« Roasted Salmon and Asparagus, page 89

**EXTRA-VIRGIN
|OLIVE OIL**

**RED BELL
PEPPER**

GARLIC

DAIRY-FREE
GLUTEN-FREE
NUT-FREE
ONE POT

Shrimp Scampi

SERVES 4 / PREP TIME 10 MINUTES / COOK TIME 15 MINUTES

*Buying frozen peeled shrimp with the tails already removed makes
this meal a snap to prepare. I prefer wild-caught shrimp to farmed
shrimp, which are more likely to have contaminants. Serve it with
cooked whole-wheat pasta, zucchini "noodles," over rice or quinoa,
or on a bed of greens for a yummy meal.*

¼ CUP EXTRA-VIRGIN OLIVE OIL

1 ONION, FINELY CHOPPED

1 RED BELL PEPPER, CHOPPED

**1½ POUNDS SHRIMP, PEELED
AND TAILS REMOVED**

6 GARLIC CLOVES, MINCED

JUICE OF 2 LEMONS

ZEST OF 2 LEMONS

½ TEASPOON SEA SALT

**⅛ TEASPOON FRESHLY GROUND
BLACK PEPPER**

1. In a large nonstick skillet over medium-high heat, heat the olive oil until
it shimmers.

2. Add the onion and red bell pepper. Cook for about 6 minutes, stirring
occasionally, until soft.

3. Add the shrimp and cook for about 5 minutes until pink.

4. Add the garlic. Cook for 30 seconds, stirring constantly.

5. Add the lemon juice and zest, salt, and pepper. Simmer for 3 minutes.

VARIATION TIP: Looking for a little color, herbal flavor, or heat? Add ¼ cup
chopped fresh Italian parsley leaves or a pinch of red pepper flakes (or both!)
just before serving.

PER SERVING Calories: 345; Total Fat: 16; Total Carbs: 10g; Sugar: 3g; Fiber: 1g;
Protein: 40g; Sodium: 424mg

Shrimp with Spicy Spinach

SERVES 4 / PREP TIME 10 MINUTES / COOK TIME 15 MINUTES

This simple one-pot meal—shrimp on a bed of cooked spinach—is a surprising complementary combination. This recipe uses Sriracha sauce, which has a little sugar in it. If you are concerned about the sugar, replace it with one chopped red chile pepper (you decide how hot you want it!) or ¼ to ½ teaspoon red pepper flakes.

¼ CUP EXTRA-VIRGIN OLIVE OIL, DIVIDED

1½ POUNDS PEELED SHRIMP

1 TEASPOON SEA SALT, DIVIDED

4 CUPS FRESH BABY SPINACH

6 GARLIC CLOVES, MINCED

½ CUP FRESHLY SQUEEZED ORANGE JUICE

1 TABLESPOON SRIRACHA SAUCE

⅛ TEASPOON FRESHLY GROUND BLACK PEPPER

1. In a large nonstick skillet over medium-high heat, heat 2 tablespoons of the olive oil until it shimmers.

2. Add the shrimp and ½ teaspoon salt. Cook for about 4 minutes, stirring occasionally, until the shrimp are pink. Transfer the shrimp to a plate, tent with aluminum foil to keep warm, and set aside.

3. Return the skillet to the heat and heat the remaining 2 tablespoons of olive oil until it shimmers.

4. Add the spinach. Cook for 3 minutes, stirring.

5. Add the garlic. Cook for 30 seconds, stirring constantly.

6. In a small bowl, whisk the orange juice, Sriracha, remaining ½ teaspoon of salt, and pepper. Add this to the spinach and cook for 3 minutes. Serve the shrimp with the spinach on the side.

PER SERVING Calories: 317; Total Fat: 16; Total Carbs: 7g; Sugar: 3g; Fiber: <1g; Protein: 38g; Sodium: 911mg

EXTRA-VIRGIN OLIVE OIL

SPINACH

GARLIC

DAIRY-FREE

GLUTEN-FREE

NUT-FREE

ONE POT

EXTRA-VIRGIN OLIVE OIL

CINNAMON

DAIRY-FREE
GLUTEN-FREE
NUT-FREE
ONE POT

Shrimp with Cinnamon Sauce

SERVES 4 / PREP TIME 10 MINUTES / COOK TIME 10 MINUTES

Shrimp and cinnamon? I know. I was skeptical, too, but one day when I was out of the spices I usually use, I tossed some cinnamon in instead and it was delicious! Cinnamon is a nice complement to the slight sweetness of the shrimp and the bite of the mustard in the sauce.

2 TABLESPOONS EXTRA-VIRGIN OLIVE OIL

1½ POUNDS PEELED SHRIMP

2 TABLESPOONS DIJON MUSTARD

1 CUP NO-SALT-ADDED CHICKEN BROTH

1 TEASPOON GROUND CINNAMON

1 TEASPOON ONION POWDER

½ TEASPOON SEA SALT

¼ TEASPOON FRESHLY GROUND BLACK PEPPER

1. In a large nonstick skillet over medium-high heat, heat the olive oil until it shimmers.

2. Add the shrimp. Cook for about 4 minutes, stirring occasionally, until the shrimp is opaque.

3. In a small bowl, whisk the mustard, chicken broth, cinnamon, onion powder, salt, and pepper. Pour this into the skillet and continue to cook for 3 minutes, stirring occasionally.

VARIATION TIP: For an even more interesting spice profile, replace the cinnamon with 1 teaspoon Chinese five-spice powder (one of my favorite spice blends).

PER SERVING Calories: 270; Total Fat: 11g; Total Carbs: 4g; Sugar: <1g; Fiber: <1g; Protein: 39g; Sodium: 664mg

THE EASY ANTI-INFLAMMATORY DIET

Pan-Seared Scallops with Lemon-Ginger Vinaigrette

SERVES 4 / PREP TIME 10 MINUTES / COOK TIME 7 MINUTES

Serve these scallops alongside a salad or on top of a bed of Citrus Spinach (page 44) for a full meal. Scallops are really fast to sear and have a sweet, briny flavor that isn't fishy at all. Spoon the vinaigrette over the scallops as well as over any greens you might be serving. It's a tangy dish you're sure to enjoy.

2 TABLESPOONS EXTRA-VIRGIN OLIVE OIL

1½ POUNDS SEA SCALLOPS

½ TEASPOON SEA SALT

⅛ TEASPOON FRESHLY GROUND BLACK PEPPER

¼ CUP LEMON-GINGER VINAIGRETTE (PAGE 153)

4. In a large nonstick skillet over medium-high heat, heat the olive oil until it shimmers.

5. Season the scallops with salt and pepper and add them to the skillet. Cook for about 3 minutes per side until just opaque.

6. Serve with the vinaigrette spooned over the top.

INGREDIENT TIP: Use sea scallops (the large ones) not bay scallops (tiny round ones) for this dish. The scallops should be pearly and have a fresh, briny (not fishy) scent. Remove the tendon on the side with a sharp knife and discard it (or freeze it to use for making fish stock). Pat them dry with a paper towel before seasoning to get a really good sear.

PER SERVING Calories: 280; Total Fat: 16; Total Carbs: 5g; Sugar: <1g; Fiber: 0g; Protein: 29g; Sodium: 508mg

EXTRA-VIRGIN OLIVE OIL

GARLIC

GINGER

DAIRY-FREE
GLUTEN-FREE
NUT-FREE

Manhattan-Style Salmon Chowder

SERVES 4 / PREP TIME 10 MINUTES / COOK TIME 15 MINUTES

Manhattan-style chowder is the less popular chowder—the red stuff. But I really like red (tomato-based) sauces with seafood, so to me this is a really great way to eat salmon. The hearty flavor of the salmon holds up well with the tomatoes in this rich chowder. Feel free to add your own veggie choices—carrots, celery, or anything else that catches your fancy. A little basil is good (¼ cup freshly chopped basil leaves), too, just before you serve it.

EXTRA-VIRGIN OLIVE OIL

RED BELL PEPPERS

SALMON

TOMATOES

DAIRY-FREE
GLUTEN-FREE
NUT-FREE
ONE POT

¼ CUP EXTRA-VIRGIN OLIVE OIL

1 RED BELL PEPPER, CHOPPED

1 POUND SKINLESS SALMON, PIN BONES REMOVED, CHOPPED INTO ½-INCH PIECES

2 (28-OUNCE) CANS CRUSHED TOMATOES, 1 DRAINED AND 1 UNDRAINED

6 CUPS NO-SALT-ADDED CHICKEN BROTH

2 CUPS DICED (½ INCH) SWEET POTATOES

1 TEASPOON ONION POWDER

½ TEASPOON SEA SALT

¼ TEASPOON FRESHLY GROUND BLACK PEPPER

1. In a large pot over medium-high heat, heat the olive oil until it shimmers.

2. Add the red bell pepper and salmon. Cook for about 5 minutes, stirring occasionally, until the fish is opaque and the bell pepper is soft.

3. Stir in the tomatoes, chicken broth, sweet potatoes, onion powder, salt, and pepper. Bring to a simmer and reduce the heat to medium. Cook for about 10 minutes, stirring occasionally, until the sweet potatoes are soft.

INGREDIENT TIP: Everybody has kitchen tweezers, right? I know, probably not. However, if you plan to eat a lot of fresh fish (and why wouldn't you?), a pair of tweezers is invaluable for picking out pin bones in salmon and other fish. Any tweezers will do, just make sure they are dedicated for kitchen use.

PER SERVING Calories: 570; Total Fat: 42; Total Carbs: 55g; Sugar: 24g; Fiber: 16g; Protein: 41g; Sodium: 1,249mg

Roasted Salmon and Asparagus

SERVES 4 / PREP TIME 5 MINUTES / COOK TIME 15 MINUTES

This easy meal comes together quickly with almost no prep time, so it's a great nutritious meal for busy weeknights. Lemon zest adds flavor to both the salmon and the asparagus.

1 POUND ASPARAGUS SPEARS, TRIMMED

2 TABLESPOONS EXTRA-VIRGIN OLIVE OIL

1 TEASPOON SEA SALT, DIVIDED

1½ POUND SALMON, CUT INTO FOUR FILLETS

⅛ TEASPOON FRESHLY CRACKED BLACK PEPPER

ZEST AND SLICES FROM 1 LEMON

1. Preheat the oven to 425°F.

2. Toss the asparagus with the olive oil and ½ teaspoon of the salt. Spread in a single layer in the bottom of a roasting pan.

3. Season the salmon with the pepper and remaining ½ teaspoon of salt. Place skin-side down on top of the asparagus.

4. Sprinkle the salmon and asparagus with the lemon zest and place the lemon slices over the fish.

5. Roast in the preheated oven 12 to 15 minutes, until the flesh is opaque.

PER SERVING Calories: 308; Total Fat: 18g; Total Carbs: 5g; Sugar: 2g; Fiber: 2g; Protein: 36g; Sodium: 545mg

EXTRA-VIRGIN OLIVE OIL

SALMON

DAIRY-FREE
GLUTEN-FREE
NUT-FREE
ONE POT

Citrus Salmon on a Bed of Greens

SERVES 4 / PREP TIME 10 MINUTES / COOK TIME 19 MINUTES

Citrus-laced salmon and greens is a lively combination. In this recipe, the citrus is lemon, but you can use lime, orange, or even grapefruit if you wish.

EXTRA-VIRGIN OLIVE OIL

SALMON

GARLIC

DAIRY-FREE
GLUTEN-FREE
NUT-FREE
ONE POT

¼ CUP EXTRA-VIRGIN OLIVE OIL, DIVIDED

1½ POUNDS SALMON

1 TEASPOON SEA SALT, DIVIDED

½ TEASPOON FRESHLY GROUND BLACK PEPPER, DIVIDED

ZEST OF 1 LEMON

6 CUPS STEMMED AND CHOPPED SWISS CHARD

3 GARLIC CLOVES, MINCED

JUICE OF 2 LEMONS

1. In a large nonstick skillet over medium-high heat, heat 2 tablespoons of the olive oil until it shimmers.

2. Season the salmon with ½ teaspoon of the salt, ¼ teaspoon of the pepper, and the lemon zest. Add the salmon to the skillet, skin-side up, and cook for about 7 minutes until the flesh is opaque. Flip the salmon and cook for 3 to 4 minutes to crisp the skin. Set aside on a plate, tented with aluminum foil.

3. Return the skillet to the heat, add the remaining 2 tablespoons of olive oil, and heat it until it shimmers.

4. Add the Swiss chard. Cook for about 7 minutes, stirring occasionally, until soft.

5. Add the garlic. Cook for 30 seconds, stirring constantly.

6. Sprinkle in the lemon juice, the remaining ½ teaspoon of salt, and the remaining ¼ teaspoon of pepper. Cook for 2 minutes.

7. Serve the salmon on the Swiss chard.

INGREDIENT TIP: Minced garlic burns easily and burned garlic is bitter. It only takes a slight amount of heat to release garlic's fragrance and flavor. The constant stirring keeps it from remaining in contact with the pan's surface for too long, which also prevents it from burning.

PER SERVING Calories: 363; Total Fat: 25; Total Carbs: 3g; Sugar: <1g; Fiber: 1g; Protein: 34g; Sodium: 662mg

THE EASY ANTI-INFLAMMATORY DIET

Orange and Maple-Glazed Salmon

SERVES 4 / PREP TIME 15 MINUTES / COOK TIME 15 MINUTES

A few years ago I discovered orange and maple have a natural kinship for salmon. The flavors go fantastically well together. A simple citrus juicer (found at any grocery store) is a great way to extract the small amounts of fresh juices these recipes use, so it's a worthwhile investment that allows you to extract more juice from the fruits than squeezing alone.

GARLIC

SALMON

DAIRY-FREE
NUT-FREE

JUICE OF 2 ORANGES

ZEST OF 1 ORANGE

¼ CUP PURE MAPLE SYRUP

2 TABLESPOONS LOW-SODIUM
SOY SAUCE

1 TEASPOON GARLIC POWDER

4 (4- TO 6-OUNCE) SALMON FILLETS,
PIN BONES REMOVED

1. Preheat the oven to 400°F.

2. In a small, shallow dish, whisk the orange juice and zest, maple syrup, soy sauce, and garlic powder.

3. Put the salmon pieces, flesh-side down, into the dish. Let it marinate for 10 minutes.

4. Transfer the salmon, skin-side up, to a rimmed baking sheet and bake for about 15 minutes until the flesh is opaque.

INGREDIENT TIP: If you wish, make a fresh batch of glaze and simmer it on the stove top until it thickens. Brush it over the salmon as it comes out of the oven for an even more orangey, mapley salmon dish.

PER SERVING Calories: 297; Total Fat: 11; Total Carbs: 18g; Sugar: 15g; Fiber: <1g; Protein: 34g; Sodium: 528mg

SALMON

TOMATOES

EXTRA-VIRGIN
OLIVE OIL

DAIRY-FREE
GLUTEN-FREE
NUT-FREE
ONE POT

Salmon Ceviche

SERVES 4 / PREP TIME 10 MINUTES, PLUS 20 MINUTES RESTING TIME

Since the salmon isn't technically cooked here (the citrus juice "cooks" it with acidity), use the freshest, best-quality salmon you can find. If you are uncomfortable with uncooked salmon, poach it lightly before adding it to the ceviche.

1 POUND SALMON, SKIN AND PIN BONES REMOVED, CUT INTO BITE-SIZE PIECES (REMOVE ANY GRAY FLESH)

½ CUP FRESHLY SQUEEZED LIME JUICE

2 TOMATOES, DICED

¼ CUP FRESH CILANTRO LEAVES, CHOPPED

1 JALAPEÑO PEPPER, SEEDED AND DICED

2 TABLESPOONS EXTRA-VIRGIN OLIVE OIL

½ TEASPOON SEA SALT

1. In a medium bowl, stir together the salmon and lime juice. Let it marinate for 20 minutes.

2. Stir in the tomatoes, cilantro, jalapeño, olive oil, and salt.

VARIATION TIP: Add some chopped red onion (about ½ onion) or some minced garlic (2 cloves).

PER SERVING Calories: 222; Total Fat: 14g; Total Carbs: 3g; Sugar: 2g; Fiber: <1g; Protein: 23g; Sodium: 288mg

Cod with Ginger and Black Beans

SERVES 4 / PREP TIME 10 MINUTES / COOK TIME 15 MINUTES

I live in the Pacific Northwest where fresh fish is abundant. If cod isn't readily available in your local grocery store or if you live away from the coasts, feel free to substitute any white-fleshed fish that is available.

2 TABLESPOONS EXTRA-VIRGIN OLIVE OIL

4 (6-OUNCE) COD FILLETS

1 TABLESPOON GRATED FRESH GINGER

1 TEASPOON SEA SALT, DIVIDED

¼ TEASPOON FRESHLY GROUND BLACK PEPPER

5 GARLIC CLOVES, MINCED

1 (14-OUNCE) CAN BLACK BEANS, DRAINED

¼ CUP CHOPPED FRESH CILANTRO LEAVES

EXTRA-VIRGIN
OLIVE OIL

GINGER

GARLIC

DAIRY-FREE
GLUTEN-FREE
NUT-FREE
ONE POT

1. In a large nonstick skillet over medium-high heat, heat the olive oil until it shimmers.

2. Season the cod with the ginger, ½ teaspoon of the salt, and the pepper. Place it in the hot oil and cook for about 4 minutes per side until the fish is opaque. Remove the cod from the pan and set it aside on a platter, tented with aluminum foil.

3. Return the skillet to the heat and add the garlic. Cook for 30 seconds, stirring constantly.

4. Stir in the black beans and the remaining ½ teaspoon of salt. Cook for 5 minutes, stirring occasionally.

5. Stir in the cilantro and spoon the black beans over the cod.

VARIATION TIP: Add ¼ cup freshly squeezed lime juice to the black beans and serve with lime wedges as a garnish to add some acidity to this dish.

PER SERVING Calories: 419; Total Fat: 2g; Total Carbs: 33g; Sugar: 1g; Fiber: 8g; Protein: 50g; Sodium: 605mg

Rosemary-Lemon Cod

SERVES 4 / PREP TIME 10 MINUTES / COOK TIME 11 MINUTES

A popular cod recipe is lemon-pepper cod, which uses lots of black pepper and lemon juice. This version adds rosemary, which has a resinous note that makes the cod and lemon pop. It's also easy to make—you'll have it on the table in about 20 minutes.

EXTRA-VIRGIN OLIVE OIL

ROSEMARY

DAIRY-FREE
GLUTEN-FREE
NUT-FREE
ONE POT

2 TABLESPOONS EXTRA-VIRGIN OLIVE OIL

1½ POUNDS COD, SKIN AND BONES REMOVED, CUT INTO 4 FILLETS

1 TABLESPOON CHOPPED FRESH ROSEMARY LEAVES

½ TEASPOON FRESHLY GROUND BLACK PEPPER, OR MORE TO TASTE

½ TEASPOON SEA SALT

JUICE OF 1 LEMON

1. In a large nonstick skillet over medium-high heat, heat the olive oil until it shimmers.

2. Season the cod with the rosemary, pepper, and salt. Add the fish to the skillet and cook for 3 to 5 minutes per side until opaque.

3. Pour the lemon juice over the cod fillets and cook for 1 minute.

PER SERVING Calories: 246; Total Fat: 9g; Total Carbs: 1g; Sugar: <1g; Fiber: <1g; Protein: 39g; Sodium: 370mg

THE EASY ANTI-INFLAMMATORY DIET

Halibut Curry

SERVES 4 / PREP TIME 10 MINUTES / COOK TIME 10 MINUTES

Halibut is abundant here in the Pacific Northwest due to our proximity to Alaska. Substitute white-fleshed saltwater fish available in your area if halibut isn't or if it's too expensive. If you're allergic to fish, use shrimp or bay scallops. Feel free to add veggies to this curry as well. Sweet potatoes, red bell peppers, onions, and carrots are all good choices.

2 TABLESPOONS EXTRA-VIRGIN OLIVE OIL

2 TEASPOONS GROUND TURMERIC

2 TEASPOONS CURRY POWDER

1½ POUNDS HALIBUT, SKIN AND BONES REMOVED, CUT INTO 1-INCH PIECES

4 CUPS NO-SALT-ADDED CHICKEN BROTH

1 (14-OUNCE) CAN LITE COCONUT MILK

½ TEASPOON SEA SALT

¼ TEASPOON FRESHLY GROUND BLACK PEPPER

1. In a large nonstick skillet over medium-high, heat the olive oil until it shimmers.

2. Add the turmeric and curry powder. Cook for 2 minutes, stirring constantly, to bloom the spices.

3. Add the halibut, chicken broth, coconut milk, salt, and pepper. Bring to a simmer and reduce the heat to medium. Simmer for 6 to 7 minutes, stirring occasionally, until the fish is opaque.

PER SERVING Calories: 429; Total Fat: 47g; Total Carbs: 5g; Sugar: <1g; Fiber: <1g; Protein: 27g; Sodium: 507mg

EXTRA-VIRGIN OLIVE OIL

TURMERIC

DAIRY-FREE
GLUTEN-FREE
ONE POT

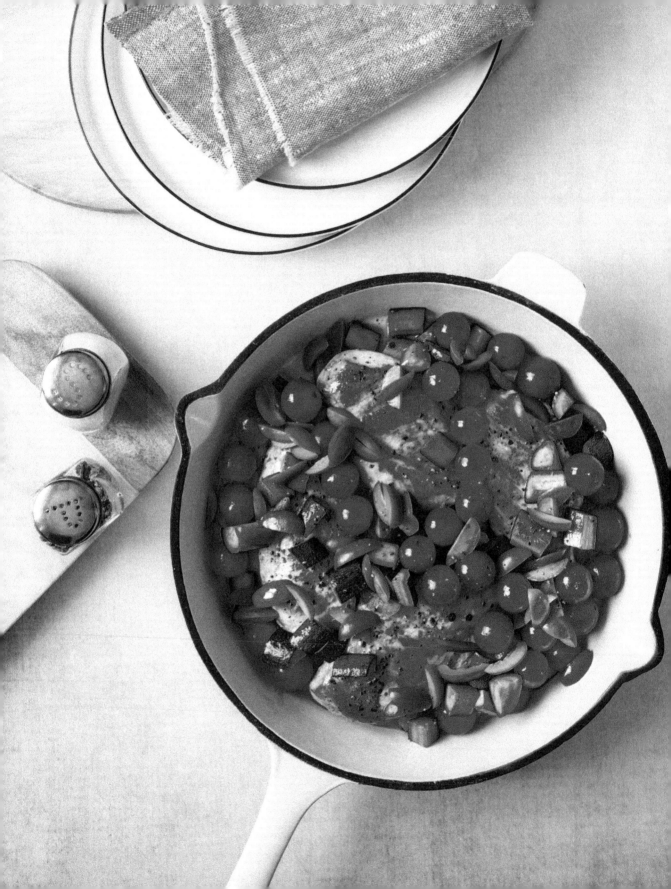

7

POULTRY DISHES

‹‹ Tuscan Chicken, page 98

GARLIC

EXTRA-VIRGIN
OLIVE OIL

TOMATOES

DAIRY-FREE
GLUTEN-FREE
NUT-FREE
ONE POT

Tuscan Chicken

SERVES 4 / PREP TIME 5 MINUTES / COOK TIME 20 MINUTES

Make a quick pan sauce to go with the chicken breasts for an easy meal. To ensure even and quicker cooking time, lightly pound half-chicken breasts to an even ½- to ¾-inch thickness between to pieces of plastic wrap or parchment paper.

4 BONELESS, SKINLESS CHICKEN BREAST HALVES, POUNDED TO ½- TO ¾-INCH THICKNESS

½ TEASPOON SEA SALT

⅛ TEASPOON FRESHLY GROUND BLACK PEPPER

1 TEASPOON GARLIC POWDER

2 TABLESPOONS EXTRA-VIRGIN OLIVE OIL

1 ZUCCHINI, CHOPPED

2 CUPS CHERRY TOMATOES

½ CUP SLICED GREEN OLIVES

¼ CUP DRY WHITE WINE

1. Season the chicken breasts with the salt, pepper, and garlic powder.

2. In a large nonstick skillet over medium-high heat, heat the olive oil until it shimmers. Add the chicken and cook 7 to 10 minutes per side, until it reaches an internal temperature of 165°F. Remove the chicken and set aside on a platter, tented with foil.

3. In the same skillet, add the zucchini, tomatoes, and olives. Cook for about 4 minutes, stirring occasionally, until the zucchini is tender.

4. Add the white wine and use a wooden spoon to scrape any browned bits from the bottom of the pan. Simmer for 1 minute. Return the chicken and any juices that have collected on the platter to the pan and stir to coat with the sauce and vegetables.

PER SERVING Calories: 171; Total Fat: 11g; Total Carbs: 8g; Sugar: 4g; Fiber: 2g; Protein: 8g; Sodium: 743mg

Chicken Cacciatore

SERVES 4 / PREP TIME 10 MINUTES / COOK TIME 20 MINUTES

This isn't technically chicken cacciatore, which involves whole pieces of chicken, but the flavor profiles are similar. You'll get double olive goodness with extra-virgin olive oil and black olives in this dish. Cutting the chicken into bite-size pieces means it cooks much more quickly. Serve over brown rice or whole-wheat pasta, or alongside a simple salad.

2 TABLESPOONS EXTRA-VIRGIN OLIVE OIL

1½ POUNDS BONELESS SKINLESS CHICKEN BREASTS, CUT INTO BITE-SIZE PIECES

2 (28-OUNCE) CANS CRUSHED TOMATOES, DRAINED

½ CUP BLACK OLIVES, CHOPPED

1 TEASPOON GARLIC POWDER

1 TEASPOON ONION POWDER

½ TEASPOON SEA SALT

⅛ TEASPOON FRESHLY GROUND BLACK PEPPER

EXTRA-VIRGIN OLIVE OIL

TOMATOES

GARLIC

DAIRY-FREE
GLUTEN-FREE
NUT-FREE
ONE POT

1. In a large nonstick skillet over medium-high heat, heat the olive oil until it shimmers.

2. Add the chicken and cook for 7 to 10 minutes, stirring occasionally, until it is browned.

3. Stir in the tomatoes, olives, garlic powder, onion powder, salt, and pepper. Simmer for 10 minutes, stirring occasionally.

VARIATION TIP: Chop ¼ cup fresh basil leaves and stir them in just before serving for a fresh, herbal flavor.

PER SERVING Calories: 305; Total Fat: 11g; Total Carbs: 34g; Sugar: 23g; Fiber: 13g; Protein: 19g; Sodium: 1,171mg

EXTRA-VIRGIN
OLIVE OIL

TURMERIC

GARLIC

DAIRY-FREE
GLUTEN-FREE
NUT-FREE
ONE POT

Chicken Adobo

SERVES 4 / PREP TIME 10 MINUTES / COOK TIME 15 MINUTES

The first time I heard of turmeric was in the 1980s in a recipe for chicken adobo. I was dubious, but I gave it a try, and it turned me into a convert. If you'd like to add some veggies to this, bell pepper works well. Choose your favorite color, remove the seeds, chop it, and add it when you cook the chicken. The black pepper in this recipe helps your body absorb the curcumin in the turmeric, so it's a great combination of spices. Serve this with steamed brown rice.

3 TABLESPOONS EXTRA-VIRGIN OLIVE OIL

1½ POUNDS BONELESS SKINLESS CHICKEN BREASTS, CUT INTO BITE-SIZE PIECES

2 TEASPOONS GROUND TURMERIC

¼ CUP LOW-SODIUM SOY SAUCE

1 TEASPOON GARLIC POWDER

1 TEASPOON ONION POWDER

½ TEASPOON SEA SALT

¼ TEASPOON FRESHLY GROUND BLACK PEPPER

1. In a large nonstick skillet over medium-high heat, heat the olive oil until it shimmers.

2. Add the chicken and turmeric. Cook for 7 to 10 minutes, stirring occasionally, until the chicken is cooked through.

3. Stir in the soy sauce, garlic powder, onion powder, salt, and pepper. Cook for 3 minutes, stirring.

INGREDIENT TIP: Let's talk about freshly ground black pepper. While it's not a requirement in these recipes, grinding black peppercorns fresh produces a lot more flavor. Plus, grinding pepper makes your cooking feel more immediate, like you're a celebrity chef prepping food on TV. You can even find peppercorns in a disposable grinder in the spice aisle of your local grocery store.

PER SERVING Calories: 698; Total Fat: 52g; Total Carbs: 11g; Sugar: 2g; Fiber: 2g; Protein: 46g; Sodium: 776mg

THE EASY ANTI-INFLAMMATORY DIET

Chicken and Bell Pepper Sauté

SERVES 4 / PREP TIME 15 MINUTES / COOK TIME 15 MINUTES

Fast and easy is the name of the game with this dish, but it's also one your family will enjoy. Serve it with steamed brown rice or roasted sweet potatoes and a simple salad for a fast anti-inflammatory supper. You can switch up the bell pepper colors if there's one more to your liking.

3 TABLESPOONS EXTRA-VIRGIN OLIVE OIL

1 RED BELL PEPPER, CHOPPED

1 ONION, CHOPPED

1½ POUNDS BONELESS, SKINLESS CHICKEN BREASTS, CUT INTO BITE-SIZE PIECES

5 GARLIC CLOVES, MINCED

½ TEASPOON SEA SALT

¼ TEASPOON FRESHLY GROUND BLACK PEPPER

1. In a large nonstick skillet over medium-high heat, heat the olive oil until it shimmers.

2. Add the red bell pepper, onion, and chicken. Cook for 10 minutes, stirring it occasionally.

3. Add the garlic, salt, and pepper. Cook for 30 seconds, stirring constantly.

INGREDIENT TIP: Remember, smaller pieces cook faster. Cut the chicken and veggies into same-size pieces (½ to 1 inch) so they cook evenly.

PER SERVING Calories: 179; Total Fat: 13g; Total Carbs: 6g; Sugar: 3g; Fiber: 1g; Protein: 10g; Sodium: 265mg

EXTRA-VIRGIN OLIVE OIL

RED BELL PEPPER

GARLIC

DAIRY-FREE
GLUTEN-FREE
NUT-FREE
ONE POT

**EXTRA-VIRGIN
OLIVE OIL**

BROCCOLI

GARLIC

GINGER

DAIRY-FREE
NUT-FREE
ONE POT

Chicken Stir-Fry

SERVES 4 / PREP TIME 15 MINUTES / COOK TIME 15 MINUTES

Every once in a while, I get in a groove when all I want is garlic, ginger, and soy sauce. When I'm in one of those moods, this dish makes the rotation. The Stir-Fry Sauce (page 149) offers a combination of flavors that makes this chicken dish better than take-out.

3 TABLESPOONS EXTRA-VIRGIN OLIVE OIL

6 SCALLIONS, WHITE AND GREEN PARTS, CHOPPED

1 CUP BROCCOLI FLORETS

1 POUND BONELESS, SKINLESS CHICKEN BREASTS, CUT INTO BITE-SIZE PIECES

1 RECIPE STIR-FRY SAUCE (PAGE 149)

TABLESPOONS TOASTED SESAME SEEDS (OPTIONAL)

1. In a large nonstick skillet over medium-high heat, heat the olive oil until it shimmers.

2. Add the scallions, broccoli, and chicken. Cook for 5 to 7 minutes, stirring occasionally, until the chicken is cooked and the vegetables are tender.

3. Add the stir-fry sauce. Cook for 5 minutes, stirring, until the sauce reduces.

4. Garnish with sesame seeds, if using.

PREPARATION TIP: For a thicker stir-fry sauce, whisk 1 tablespoon arrowroot powder (or cornstarch) into the sauce before adding it to the pan. Cook, stirring constantly, just until the sauce thickens.

PER SERVING Calories: 363; Total Fat: 22g; Total Carbs: 7g; Sugar: 2g; Fiber: 2g; Protein: 36g; Sodium: 993mg

THE EASY ANTI-INFLAMMATORY DIET

Chicken Salad Sandwiches

SERVES 4 / PREP TIME 10 MINUTES

Sometimes you just want a sandwich. If you plan to make this as a meal to take with you, I recommend storing the chicken salad separately from the bread and assembling the sandwich just before you eat it so the bread doesn't get soggy. If you can't have gluten, do what I do and make these as lettuce wraps.

2 CUPS CHOPPED, COOKED, SKINLESS CHICKEN FROM A ROTISSERIE CHICKEN

¼ CUP ANTI-INFLAMMATORY MAYONNAISE (PAGE 148)

1 RED BELL PEPPER, MINCED

2 TABLESPOONS CHOPPED FRESH TARRAGON LEAVES

2 TEASPOONS DIJON MUSTARD

½ TEASPOON SEA SALT

8 SLICES WHOLE-WHEAT BREAD

1. In a medium bowl, stir together the chicken, mayonnaise, red bell pepper, tarragon, mustard, and salt.

2. Spread on 4 slices of bread and top with the remaining bread.

VARIATION TIP: Omit the tarragon and replace it with ¼ cup chopped fresh fennel and 2 tablespoons chopped fresh fennel fronds.

PER SERVING (1 SANDWICH) Calories: 315; Total Fat: 9g; Total Carbs: 30g; Sugar: 6g; Fiber: 4g; Protein: 28g; Sodium: 677mg

EXTRA-VIRGIN OLIVE OIL

RED BELL PEPPER

DAIRY-FREE

NUT-FREE

ONE POT

Easy Chicken and Broccoli

SERVES 4 / PREP TIME 10 MINUTES / COOK TIME 7 MINUTES

There's not a lot to this recipe, so feel free to spice it up any way you want with extra veggies (try bell peppers or carrots), herbs (thyme and rosemary are both nice), or by changing your protein (chopped tofu, shrimp, or ground beef all work well). The beauty of this recipe is its simplicity.

EXTRA-VIRGIN
OLIVE OIL

BROCCOLI

GARLIC

DAIRY-FREE
GLUTEN-FREE
NUT-FREE
ONE POT

3 TABLESPOONS EXTRA-VIRGIN OLIVE OIL

1½ POUNDS BONELESS, SKINLESS CHICKEN BREASTS, CUT INTO BITE-SIZE PIECES

1½ CUPS BROCCOLI FLORETS, OR CHOPPED BROCCOLI STEMS

½ ONION, CHOPPED

½ TEASPOON SEA SALT

⅛ TEASPOON FRESHLY GROUND BLACK PEPPER

3 GARLIC CLOVES, MINCED

2 CUPS COOKED BROWN RICE

1. In a large nonstick skillet over medium-high heat, heat the olive oil until it shimmers.

2. Add the chicken, broccoli, onion, salt, and pepper. Cook for about 7 minutes, stirring occasionally, until the chicken is cooked.

3. Add the garlic. Cook for 30 seconds, stirring constantly.

4. Toss with the brown rice to serve.

PER SERVING Calories: 345; Total Fat: 14g; Total Carbs: 41g; Sugar: 1g; Fiber: 3g; Protein: 14g; Sodium: 276mg

Rosemary Chicken

SERVES 4 / PREP TIME 10 MINUTES / COOK TIME 20 MINUTES

Chicken and rosemary just belong together. This main course is a fragrant centerpiece to a meal that can include a simple salad or steamed veggies.

1½ POUNDS CHICKEN BREAST TENDERS

2 TABLESPOONS EXTRA-VIRGIN OLIVE OIL

2 TABLESPOONS CHOPPED FRESH ROSEMARY LEAVES

½ TEASPOON SEA SALT

⅛ TEASPOON FRESHLY GROUND BLACK PEPPER

1. Preheat the oven to 425°F.

2. Place the chicken tenders on a rimmed baking sheet. Brush them with the olive oil and sprinkle with the rosemary, salt, and pepper.

3. Bake for 15 to 20 minutes, or until the juices run clear.

INGREDIENT TIP: So how do you get the rosemary leaves off those woody stems? Hold the bottom of the sprig between your thumb and forefinger of your nondominant hand and, with your dominant hand, starting at the top, pinch your thumb and forefinger around the woody stem, and run it down the stem. This will detach the rosemary leaves from the stems.

PER SERVING Calories: 389; Total Fat: 20g; Total Carbs: 1g; Sugar: 0g; Fiber: <1g; Protein: 49g; Sodium: 381mg

EXTRA-VIRGIN OLIVE OIL

ROSEMARY

DAIRY-FREE
GLUTEN-FREE
NUT-FREE
ONE POT

**EXTRA-VIRGIN
OLIVE OIL**

**RED BELL
PEPPER**

**DAIRY-FREE
NUT-FREE
ONE POT**

Chicken Sandwiches with Roasted Red Pepper Aioli

SERVES 4 / PREP TIME 10 MINUTES / COOK TIME 10 MINUTES

Roasted red peppers from a jar mixed with Anti-Inflammatory Mayonnaise (page 148) make a savory sauce for these sandwiches. Adding slices of red pepper doubles the flavor and inflammation-fighting benefits.

2 TABLESPOONS EXTRA-VIRGIN OLIVE OIL

1 POUND BONELESS, SKINLESS CHICKEN BREASTS, CUT INTO 4 EQUAL PIECES AND POUNDED ½ INCH THICK

½ TEASPOON SEA SALT

⅛ TEASPOON FRESHLY GROUND BLACK PEPPER

6 ROASTED RED PEPPER SLICES, DIVIDED

¼ CUP ANTI-INFLAMMATORY MAYONNAISE (PAGE 148)

4 WHOLE-WHEAT BUNS

1. In a large nonstick skillet over medium-high heat, heat the olive oil until it shimmers.

2. Season the chicken with salt and pepper. Add it to the skillet and cook for about 4 minutes per side until the juices run clear.

3. While the chicken cooks, in a blender or food processor, combine the mayonnaise and 2 red pepper pieces. Blend until smooth.

4. Spread the sauce on the buns and top with the remaining roasted red pepper slices.

5. Top with the chicken.

PER SERVING Calories: 318; Total Fat: 15g; Total Carbs: 36g; Sugar: 7g; Fiber: 6g; Protein: 13g; Sodium: 599mg

Gingered Turkey Meatballs

SERVES 4 / PREP TIME 10 MINUTES / COOK TIME 10 MINUTES

Instead of bread crumbs, I use shredded cabbage (buy bagged coleslaw mix with the cabbage preshredded) to lighten these meatballs. The ginger and aromatics add character. Making smaller meatballs means they're ready faster on the stove top.

1½ POUNDS GROUND TURKEY

1 CUP SHREDDED CABBAGE

¼ CUP CHOPPED FRESH CILANTRO LEAVES

1 TABLESPOON GRATED FRESH GINGER

1 TEASPOON GARLIC POWDER

1 TEASPOON ONION POWDER

½ TEASPOON SEA SALT

⅛ TEASPOON FRESHLY GROUND BLACK PEPPER

2 TABLESPOONS OLIVE OIL

1. In a large bowl, combine the turkey, cabbage, cilantro, ginger, garlic powder, onion powder, salt, and pepper. Mix well. Form the turkey mixture into about 20 (¾-inch) meatballs.

2. In a large nonstick skillet over medium-high heat, heat the olive oil until it shimmers.

3. Add the meatballs and cook for about 10 minutes, turning as they brown.

PREPARATION TIP: I find that when making a meat mixture for meatballs or meatloaf, stirring it with a spoon is a lesson in frustration. So I get my (clean) hands in there and mix it up that way. It allows me to feel that the ingredients are well incorporated and keeps me from overworking the meat, so it doesn't get too tough.

PER SERVING (5 MEATBALLS) Calories: 408; Total Fat: 26g; Total Carbs: 4g; Sugar: 1g; Fiber: 1g; Protein: 47g; Sodium: 426mg

GINGER

GARLIC

EXTRA-VIRGIN OLIVE OIL

DAIRY-FREE
GLUTEN-FREE
NUT-FREE
ONE POT

EXTRA-VIRGIN OLIVE OIL

ROSEMARY

DAIRY-FREE
NUT-FREE
ONE POT

Turkey Scaloppine with Rosemary and Lemon Sauce

SERVES 4 / PREP TIME 10 MINUTES / COOK TIME 15 MINUTES

Scaloppine is a way of describing a turkey cutlet you pound the heck out of until it's super thin (see Tip). It cooks quickly, and that's a good thing when you don't have much time to spend in the kitchen. You'll need to work in batches, cooking each piece separately. But because each piece cooks in three to four minutes, you'll be enjoying your meal in no time flat.

¼ CUP WHOLE-WHEAT FLOUR

1 TEASPOON SEA SALT, DIVIDED

¼ TEASPOON FRESHLY GROUND BLACK PEPPER

4¼ TO 4½ POUNDS BONELESS, SKINLESS TURKEY BREAST CUTLETS, POUNDED ¼ INCH THICK

¼ CUP EXTRA-VIRGIN OLIVE OIL, DIVIDED

JUICE OF 3 LEMONS

ZEST OF 1 LEMON

1 TABLESPOON CHOPPED FRESH ROSEMARY LEAVES

1. Preheat the oven to 200°F.

2. Line a baking sheet with parchment paper.

3. In a shallow dish, whisk the flour, ½ teaspoon salt, and the pepper.

4. Working with one piece at a time, dip each cutlet in the flour and pat off any excess.

5. In a large skillet over medium-high heat, use 1 tablespoon olive oil for each cutlet in the batch and heat until it shimmers. Add the cutlets to the hot oil and cook for about 2 minutes per side. Transfer each cutlet to the prepared baking sheet when cooked. When they are all cooked, put the baking sheet in the oven to keep them warm.

6. When all the cutlets are cooked and warming in the oven, return the skillet to the heat. Add the lemon juice and zest to the pan. Use a wooden spoon to scrape any browned bits from the bottom of the pan.

7. Add the remaining ½ teaspoon of salt and the rosemary. Cook for about 2 minutes, stirring constantly, until the sauce thickens. Serve the sauce spooned over the cutlets.

PREPARATION TIP: To pound the cutlets, you could buy a special meat-pounding mallet or you could use any kind of heavy object with a flat surface, like a rolling pin. Put the turkey pieces between two pieces of parchment. Use your pounding tool to pound the cutlets until they are ¼ inch thick.

PER SERVING Calories: 188; Total Fat: 13g; Total Carbs: 8g; Sugar: 1g; Fiber: <1g; Protein: 10g; Sodium: 478mg

**EXTRA-VIRGIN
OLIVE OIL**

KALE

GARLIC

DAIRY-FREE
GLUTEN-FREE
NUT-FREE
ONE POT

Turkey and Kale Sauté

SERVES 4 / PREP TIME 10 MINUTES / COOK TIME 10 MINUTES

Using ground turkey breast here makes this sauté a breeze on a busy night. If you'd like some variety, cook 1 cup sliced mushrooms along with the turkey, kale, and onions. You can also use 1 teaspoon dried thyme in place of the fresh thyme.

2 TABLESPOONS EXTRA-VIRGIN OLIVE OIL

1½ POUNDS GROUND TURKEY BREAST

2 CUPS STEMMED AND CHOPPED KALE

½ ONION, CHOPPED

2 TABLESPOONS FRESH THYME LEAVES

½ TEASPOON SEA SALT

⅛ TEASPOON FRESHLY GROUND BLACK PEPPER

5 GARLIC CLOVES, MINCED

1. In a large nonstick skillet over medium-high heat, heat the olive oil until it shimmers.

2. Add the turkey, kale, onion, thyme, salt, and pepper. Cook for about 5 minutes, crumbling the turkey with a spoon until it browns.

3. Add the garlic. Cook for 30 seconds, stirring constantly.

PER SERVING Calories: 413; Total Fat: 20g; Total Carbs: 7g; Sugar: <1g; Fiber: 1g; Protein: 50g; Sodium: 358mg

Turkey Burgers with Ginger-Teriyaki Sauce and Pineapple

SERVES 4 / PREP TIME 10 MINUTES / COOK TIME 10 MINUTES

Serve these burgers on whole-wheat buns, or enjoy them in a lettuce wrap with the sauce spooned over the top. Pineapple and teriyaki sauce are a sweet and savory accompaniment to these turkey burgers.

1 POUND GROUND TURKEY BREAST, FORMED INTO 4 PATTIES

½ TEASPOON SEA SALT

⅛ TEASPOON FRESHLY GROUND BLACK PEPPER

2 TABLESPOONS EXTRA-VIRGIN OLIVE OIL

1 RECIPE GINGER-TERIYAKI SAUCE (PAGE 150)

4 PINEAPPLE RINGS

1. Season the turkey burgers with salt and pepper.

2. In a large nonstick skillet over medium-high heat, heat the olive oil until it shimmers.

3. Add the burgers and cook for about 7 minutes, turning once, until cooked through and browned on both sides.

4. While the burgers cook, in a small saucepan over medium-high heat, bring the teriyaki sauce to a simmer, stirring constantly. Cook for 1 to 2 minutes until the sauce thickens.

5. Spoon the warmed sauce over the cooked burgers and top with the pineapple rings.

PER SERVING Calories: 366; Total Fat: 16g; Total Carbs: 23g; Sugar: 10g; Fiber: <1g; Protein: 34g; Sodium: 1,089mg

EXTRA-VIRGIN OLIVE OIL

GINGER

DAIRY-FREE
NUT-FREE

EXTRA-VIRGIN
OLIVE OIL

RED BELL
PEPPER

ROSEMARY

GARLIC

DAIRY-FREE
GLUTEN-FREE
NUT-FREE
ONE POT

Turkey with Bell Peppers and Rosemary

SERVES 4 / PREP TIME 10 MINUTES / COOK TIME 10 MINUTES

While this recipe calls for red bell pepper, feel free to use your favorite color. Try purple, orange, or yellow, which all have a similar mild, sweet flavor. Serve with quinoa and some steamed veggies for a complete anti-inflammatory meal.

3 TABLESPOONS EXTRA-VIRGIN OLIVE OIL

2 RED BELL PEPPERS, CHOPPED

1 ONION, CHOPPED

1½ POUNDS BONELESS, SKINLESS TURKEY BREASTS, CUT INTO BITE-SIZE PIECES

2 TABLESPOONS CHOPPED FRESH ROSEMARY LEAVES

½ TEASPOON SEA SALT

⅛ TEASPOON FRESHLY GROUND BLACK PEPPER

3 GARLIC CLOVES, MINCED

1. In a large nonstick skillet over medium-high heat, heat the olive oil until it shimmers.

2. Add the red bell peppers, onion, turkey, rosemary, salt, and pepper. Cook for 7 to 10 minutes, stirring occasionally, until the turkey is cooked and the vegetables are tender.

3. Add the garlic. Cook for 30 seconds more, stirring constantly.

VARIATION TIP: Replace the red bell peppers with 1 cup sliced mushrooms and replace the rosemary with 2 tablespoons chopped fresh thyme leaves.

PER SERVING Calories: 303; Total Fat: 14g; Total Carbs: 15g; Sugar: 10g; Fiber: 2g; Protein: 30g; Sodium: 387mg

THE EASY ANTI-INFLAMMATORY DIET

Ground Turkey and Spinach Stir-Fry

SERVES 4 / PREP TIME 10 MINUTES / COOK TIME 10 MINUTES

I like ground turkey in stir-fries because it cooks in no time at all. For a tempting side dish, stir about ½ cup coconut milk, the juice of 1 lime, 1 tablespoon of soy sauce, and 1 tablespoon of grated fresh ginger into some cooked brown rice.

2 TABLESPOONS EXTRA-VIRGIN OLIVE OIL

1½ POUNDS GROUND TURKEY BREAST

1 ONION, CHOPPED

4 CUPS FRESH BABY SPINACH

1 RECIPE STIR-FRY SAUCE (PAGE 149)

1. In a large nonstick skillet over medium-high heat, heat the olive oil until it shimmers.

2. Add the turkey, onion, and spinach. Cook for about 5 minutes, breaking up the turkey with a spoon, until the meat is browned.

3. Add the stir-fry sauce. Cook for 3 to 4 minutes, stirring constantly, until it thickens.

PER SERVING Calories: 424; Total Fat: 20g; Total Carbs: 9g; Sugar: 3g; Fiber: 2g; Protein: 51g; Sodium: 1,016mg

EXTRA-VIRGIN OLIVE OIL

SPINACH

GARLIC

GINGER

DAIRY-FREE
NUT-FREE
ONE POT

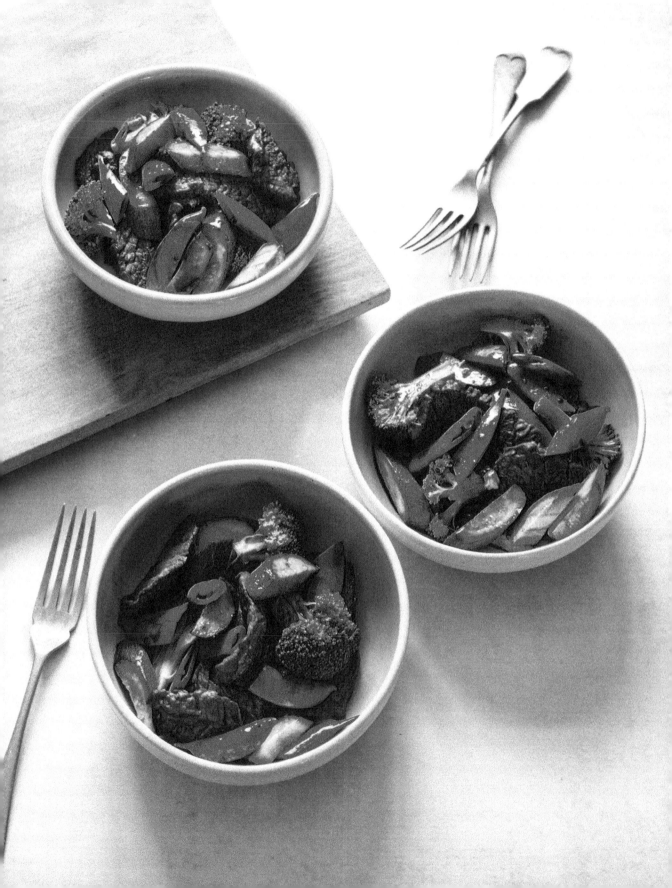

8

MEAT DISHES

<< Beef and Broccoli Stir-Fry, page 127

GARLIC

ROSEMARY

EXTRA-VIRGIN
OLIVE OIL

DAIRY-FREE
GLUTEN-FREE
NUT-FREE

Mustard and Rosemary Pork Tenderloin

SERVES 4 / PREP TIME 10 MINUTES / COOK TIME 15 MINUTES,
PLUS 5 MINUTES RESTING TIME

Pork tenderloin cooks quickly in the oven. To keep it juicy, let the meat rest for five minutes or so before you cut into it. The juices reabsorb into the meat instead of running out all over the cutting board.

½ CUP FRESH PARSLEY LEAVES

¼ CUP DIJON MUSTARD

6 GARLIC CLOVES

3 TABLESPOONS FRESH
ROSEMARY LEAVES

3 TABLESPOONS EXTRA-VIRGIN
OLIVE OIL

½ TEASPOON SEA SALT

¼ TEASPOON FRESHLY GROUND
BLACK PEPPER

1 (1½-POUND) PORK TENDERLOIN

1. Preheat the oven to 400°F.

2. In a blender or food processor, combine the parsley, mustard, garlic, rosemary, olive oil, salt, and pepper. Pulse in 1-second pulses, about 20 times, until a paste forms. Rub this paste all over the tenderloin and put the pork on a rimmed baking sheet.

3. Bake the pork for about 15 minutes, or until it registers 165°F on an instant-read meat thermometer.

4. Let rest for 5 minutes, slice, and serve.

VARIATION TIP: Use the mustard, olive oil, salt, and pepper paste base, but play with the herbs. I like the zest of a lemon, 3 tablespoons fresh thyme leaves and parsley, or the zest of 1 lime, ¼ cup fresh cilantro leaves, 3 garlic cloves, and 1 jalapeño pepper.

PER SERVING Calories: 362; Total Fat: 18g; Total Carbs: 5g; Sugar: <1g; Fiber: 2g; Protein: 2g; Sodium: 515mg

THE EASY ANTI-INFLAMMATORY DIET

Pork Chops with Gingered Applesauce

SERVES 4 / PREP TIME 10 MINUTES / COOK TIME 15 MINUTES

Pork and apples are a classic combination. Make the applesauce while the pork cooks and serve it warm, spooned over the pork chops or on the side. Add a salad or some quinoa, and you've got a quick, nutritious, anti-inflammatory meal.

4 THIN-CUT PORK CHOPS

½ TEASPOON SEA SALT

⅛ TEASPOON FRESHLY GROUND BLACK PEPPER

6 APPLES, PEELED, CORED, AND CHOPPED

¼ CUP PACKED BROWN SUGAR

¼ CUP WATER

TABLESPOON GRATED FRESH GINGER

1. Preheat the oven to 425°F.

2. Season the pork chops with the salt and pepper, put them on a rimmed baking sheet. Bake for about 15 minutes, or until the pork registers an internal temperature of 165°F on an instant-read meat thermometer.

3. Meanwhile, in a large pot over medium-high heat, stir together the apples, brown sugar, water, and ginger. Cover and cook for about 10 minutes, stirring occasionally, until the apples have cooked into a sauce.

INGREDIENT TIP: The apples you use can change the flavor and texture of your applesauce for better or worse. For this, I recommend using two varieties of sweet-tart apples, such as three Honeycrisp and three Granny Smith.

PER SERVING Calories: 442; Total Fat: 10g; Total Carbs: 56g; Sugar: 44g; Fiber: 8g; Protein: 35g; Sodium: 301mg

GINGER

DAIRY-FREE
GLUTEN-FREE
NUT-FREE

Thin-Cut Pork Chops with Mustardy Kale

SERVES 4 / PREP TIME 10 MINUTES / COOK TIME 15 MINUTES

EXTRA-VIRGIN OLIVE OIL

KALE

DAIRY-FREE
GLUTEN-FREE
NUT-FREE

I live in a house where certain adults are a bit iffy about certain vegetables—such as kale. Kale may not be everybody's favorite, but if you handle it the right way, it can be quite good. The mustard and garlic here temper this cruciferous vegetable's flavor for the better.

4 THIN-CUT PORK CHOPS

1 TEASPOON SEA SALT, DIVIDED

¼ TEASPOON FRESHLY GROUND BLACK PEPPER, DIVIDED

4 TABLESPOONS DIJON MUSTARD, DIVIDED

3 TABLESPOONS EXTRA-VIRGIN OLIVE OIL

½ RED ONION, FINELY CHOPPED

4 CUPS STEMMED AND CHOPPED KALE

2 TABLESPOONS APPLE CIDER VINEGAR

1. Preheat the oven to 425°F.

2. Season the pork chops with ½ teaspoon of the salt and ⅛ teaspoon of the pepper. Spread 2 tablespoons of the mustard over them and put them on a rimmed baking sheet. Bake for about 15 minutes, or until the pork registers an internal temperature of 165°F on an instant-read meat thermometer.

3. While the pork cooks, in a large nonstick skillet over medium-high, heat the olive oil until it shimmers.

4. Add the red onion and kale. Cook for about 7 minutes, stirring occasionally, until the vegetables soften.

5. In a small bowl, whisk the remaining 2 tablespoons of mustard, the cider vinegar, the remaining ½ teaspoon of salt, and the remaining ⅛ teaspoon of pepper. Add this to the kale. Cook for 2 minutes, stirring.

INGREDIENT TIP: Any type of vinegar works here. I like the flavor of apple cider vinegar. Another that goes well with pork is red wine vinegar, so use what you have on hand.

PER SERVING Calories: 504; Total Fat: 39g; Total Carbs: 10g; Sugar: <1g; Fiber: 2g; Protein: 28g; Sodium: 755mg

Macadamia-Dusted Pork Cutlets

SERVES 4 / PREP TIME 10 MINUTES / COOK TIME 10 MINUTES

A crust made of macadamia nuts adds a nuanced flavor to the pork. The trick here is to pound the slices of pork tenderloin quite thin so they cook quickly. Serve this with tropical fruit and some rice for an island-themed dinner.

MACADAMIA
NUTS

EXTRA-VIRGIN
OLIVE OIL

DAIRY-FREE
GLUTEN-FREE

1 (1-POUND) PORK TENDERLOIN, CUT INTO ½-INCH SLICES AND POUNDED UNIFORMLY THIN

1 TEASPOON SEA SALT, DIVIDED

¼ TEASPOON FRESHLY GROUND BLACK PEPPER, DIVIDED

½ CUP MACADAMIA NUTS, PULSED IN A BLENDER OR FOOD PROCESSOR TO FORM A POWDER

1 CUP FULL-FAT COCONUT MILK

2 TABLESPOONS EXTRA-VIRGIN OLIVE OIL

1. Preheat the oven to 400°F.

2. Season the pork chops with ½ teaspoon of the salt and ⅛ teaspoon of the pepper.

3. In a shallow dish, stir together the macadamia nut powder, the remaining ½ teaspoon of salt, and the remaining ⅛ teaspoon of pepper.

4. In another shallow dish, whisk the coconut milk and olive oil to combine.

5. Dip the pork into the coconut milk and into the macadamia nut powder. Put it on a rimmed baking sheet. Repeat with the remaining pork slices.

6. Bake the pork for about 10 minutes, or until it registers an internal temperature of 165°F measured on an instant-read meat thermometer.

PREPARATION TIP: You don't need to pound the heck out of the pork here—your goal is to pound it slightly so the pieces are a uniform width all the way across. This allows it to cook evenly in the oven.

PER SERVING Calories: 437; Total Fat: 33g; Total Carbs: 6g; Sugar: 3g; Fiber: 3g; Protein: 33g; Sodium: 309mg

EXTRA-VIRGIN OLIVE OIL

TOMATOES

GARLIC

DAIRY-FREE
GLUTEN-FREE
NUT-FREE
ONE POT

Garlicky Lamb Stew

SERVES 4 / PREP TIME 15 MINUTES / COOK TIME 15 MINUTES

Draining the ground lamb after it cooks reduces the saturated fat in this stew. I just put it in a colander in the sink and let the fat drain off for a minute or two before returning it to the pan. A little lamb fat remaining in the pan helps the veggies cook.

1 POUND GROUND LAMB

1 TABLESPOON EXTRA-VIRGIN OLIVE OIL

1 ONION, CHOPPED

1 TEASPOON DRIED OREGANO

½ TEASPOON SEA SALT

¼ TEASPOON FRESHLY GROUND BLACK PEPPER

1 (28-OUNCE) CAN CHOPPED TOMATOES, DRAINED

5 GARLIC CLOVES, MINCED

1. In a large nonstick skillet over medium-high heat, cook the lamb for about 5 minutes, crumbling it with a wooden spoon until it browns. Drain the fat and remove the lamb to a dish.

2. Return the skillet to the heat, add the olive oil, and heat it until it shimmers.

3. Add the onion, oregano, salt, and pepper. Cook for 5 minutes, stirring, until the onions are soft.

4. Return the lamb to the skillet and stir in the tomatoes. Cook for 3 minutes, stirring occasionally, or until heated through.

5. Add the garlic. Cook for 30 seconds, stirring constantly.

PER SERVING Calories: 295; Total Fat: 12g; Total Carbs: 12g; Sugar: 7g; Fiber: 3g; Protein: 34g; Sodium: 332mg

THE EASY ANTI-INFLAMMATORY DIET

Lamb Meatballs with Garlic Aioli

SERVES 4 / PREP TIME 15 MINUTES / COOK TIME 15 MINUTES

Baking the meatballs allows the fat to drain out, which minimizes the saturated fat in this recipe. If you're concerned, use ground turkey, chicken, or extra-lean ground beef. The flavor will be slightly different, but still quite satisfying.

1½ POUNDS GROUND LAMB

2 TABLESPOONS DRIED ROSEMARY LEAVES

1 TABLESPOON DRIED OREGANO

1 TEASPOON ONION POWDER

1 TEASPOON GARLIC POWDER

½ TEASPOON SEA SALT

¼ TEASPOON FRESHLY GROUND BLACK PEPPER

½ CUP GARLIC AIOLI (PAGE 151)

1. Preheat the oven to 400°F.

2. In a large bowl, mix the lamb, rosemary, oregano, onion powder, garlic powder, salt, and pepper. Roll the mixture into about 20 (¾-inch) balls and put them on a rimmed baking sheet.

3. Bake for about 15 minutes, or until the internal temperature registers 145°F on an instant-read meat thermometer.

4. Serve with the aioli.

INGREDIENT TIP: If you've got time, consider chopping fresh herbs to replace the dried. A great way to do this is to put the herb leaves in a food processor or blender and pulse in 1-second pulses until they are chopped. Fresh herbs aren't as strongly flavored as dried (seems counterintuitive, doesn't it?), so you'll need 5 garlic cloves, and 2 tablespoons each of fresh oregano and rosemary.

PER SERVING (5 MEATBALLS) Calories: 445; Total Fat: 23g; Total Carbs: 10g; Sugar: 2g; Fiber: 1g; Protein: 48g; Sodium: 574mg

ROSEMARY

GARLIC

EXTRA-VIRGIN OLIVE OIL

DAIRY-FREE
GLUTEN-FREE
NUT-FREE

EXTRA-VIRGIN
OLIVE OIL

BLUEBERRIES

GLUTEN-FREE
NUT-FREE
ONE POT

Beef Tenderloin with Savory Blueberry Sauce

SERVES 4 / PREP TIME 10 MINUTES / COOK TIME 15 MINUTES

Savory blueberry sauce? I was doubtful, too, until I tried it. In this one-pot meal, you make the sauce in the same pan in which you cook the beef. Choose beef filets or buy a beef tenderloin roast and cut it into individual steaks.

4 BEEF TENDERLOIN FILETS, ABOUT ¾ INCH THICK

1 TEASPOON SEA SALT, DIVIDED

¼ TEASPOON FRESHLY GROUND BLACK PEPPER, DIVIDED

2 TABLESPOONS EXTRA-VIRGIN OLIVE OIL

1 SHALLOT, FINELY MINCED

½ CUP TAWNY PORT

2 CUPS FRESH BLUEBERRIES

3 TABLESPOONS VERY COLD BUTTER, CUT INTO PIECES

1. Season the beef with ½ teaspoon of the salt and ⅛ teaspoon of the pepper.

2. In a large skillet over medium-high heat, heat the olive oil until it shimmers.

3. Add the seasoned steaks. Cook for about 5 minutes per side, or until the beef registers an internal temperature of 130°F on an instant-read meat thermometer. Set aside on a platter, tented with aluminum foil.

4. Return the skillet to the heat. Add the shallot, port, blueberries, and the remaining ½ teaspoon of salt, and the remaining ⅛ teaspoon of pepper. Use a wooden spoon to scrape any browned bits from the bottom of the pan. Bring to a simmer and reduce the heat to medium-low. Simmer for about 4 minutes, stirring and smashing the blueberries slightly, until the liquid reduces by half.

5. One piece at a time, whisk in the butter. Return the meat to the skillet. Turn it once to coat with the sauce. Serve with the remaining sauce spooned over the meat.

SUBSTITUTION TIP: When wild blackberries are in season in midsummer, they make a mouthwatering substitution for the blueberries. If you are concerned about the port wine, replace it with an equal amount of no-salt-added chicken broth.

PER SERVING Calories: 554; Total Fat: 32g; Total Carbs: 14g; Sugar: 8g; Fiber: 2g; Protein: 50g; Sodium: 632mg

EXTRA-VIRGIN
OLIVE OIL

GARLIC

DAIRY-FREE
GLUTEN-FREE
NUT-FREE

Beef Flank Steak Tacos with Guacamole

SERVES 4 / PREP TIME 10 MINUTES / COOK TIME 14 MINUTES,
PLUS 5 MINUTES RESTING TIME

If you have a little extra time, make the paste early and let the steak sit for three to four hours to marinate, which will up the flavor. However, it's not completely necessary for flavorful tacos. Serve this with either whole-wheat tortillas or large lettuce leaves as wraps.

¼ CUP FRESH CILANTRO LEAVES

6 TABLESPOONS EXTRA-VIRGIN OLIVE OIL, DIVIDED

4 GARLIC CLOVES, MINCED

1 JALAPEÑO PEPPER, CHOPPED

1½ POUNDS BEEF FLANK STEAK

½ TEASPOON SEA SALT

⅛ TEASPOON FRESHLY GROUND BLACK PEPPER

1 RECIPE GUACAMOLE (PAGE 48)

1. In a blender or food processor, combine the cilantro, 4 tablespoons of the olive oil, the garlic, and jalapeño. Pulse 10 to 20 (1-second) pulses to make a paste. Set aside 1 tablespoon of the paste and spread the remainder over the flank steak. Let it rest for 5 minutes.

2. In a large skillet over medium-high heat, heat the remaining 2 tablespoons of olive oil until it shimmers.

3. Add the steak. Cook for about 7 minutes per side, or until it registers an internal temperature of 125°F on an instant-read meat thermometer.

4. Transfer the steak to a cutting board and let rest for 5 minutes. Slice it against the grain into ½-inch-thick slices. Place the slices in a medium bowl and toss with the reserved 1 tablespoon of herb paste.

5. Serve with the guacamole.

VARIATION TIP: Pump up the flavor in the herb paste with 3 chopped scallions (white and green parts), ½ teaspoon chili powder, and the juice of 1 lime.

INGREDIENT TIP: What does it mean to cut beef against the grain? Take a close look at the raw steak, and you'll notice long meat (muscle) fibers running in one direction. Cut perpendicular to these fibers. This shortens the fibers, which makes the beef much more tender.

PER SERVING Calories: 717; Total Fat: 52g; Total Carbs: 12g; Sugar: 8g; Fiber: 1g; Protein: 54g; Sodium: 590mg

Ground Beef Chili with Tomatoes

SERVES 4 / PREP TIME 10 MINUTES / COOK TIME 15 MINUTES

TOMATOES

GARLIC

DAIRY-FREE
GLUTEN-FREE
NUT-FREE
ONE POT

Chili is a great option for the slow cooker. Brown the beef in a skillet, drain off any fat, and toss the meat in the slow cooker with the remaining ingredients. Cover, set on low heat, and come back eight hours later to enjoy. To brighten the flavors if you cook it in a slow cooker, stir in ¼ cup chopped fresh cilantro leaves just before serving. Or, cook it on the stove top and have dinner ready in 30 minutes.

1 POUND EXTRA-LEAN GROUND BEEF

1 ONION, CHOPPED

2 (28-OUNCE) CANS CHOPPED TOMATOES, UNDRAINED

2 (14-OUNCE) CANS KIDNEY BEANS, DRAINED

1 TABLESPOON CHILI POWDER

1 TEASPOON GARLIC POWDER

½ TEASPOON SEA SALT

1. In a large pot over medium-high heat, cook the beef and onion for about 5 minutes, crumbling the beef with a wooden spoon until it browns.

2. Stir in the tomatoes, kidney beans, chili powder, garlic powder, and salt. Bring to a simmer. Cook for 10 minutes, stirring.

VARIATION TIP: I like to make homemade chili spice, which I keep in a resealable bag in the cupboard. Instead of the garlic powder, salt, and chili powder, I add 2 tablespoons of my seasoning blend, which contains ¼ cup chili powder, 2 tablespoons dried oregano, 1 tablespoon garlic powder, 1 tablespoon onion powder, 1 tablespoon ground cumin, 1 tablespoon ground coriander, and 1 tablespoon sea salt.

PER SERVING Calories: 890; Total Fat: 20g; Total Carbs: 63g; Sugar: 13g; Fiber: 17g; Protein: 116g; Sodium: 562mg

THE EASY ANTI-INFLAMMATORY DIET

Beef and Broccoli Stir-Fry

SERVES 4 / PREP TIME 10 MINUTES / COOK TIME 10 MINUTES

This quick stir-fry is fantastic by itself, and it's also delicious served over steamed brown rice. It's best when freshly made, although it will keep in the fridge for up to three days.

2 TABLESPOONS EXTRA-VIRGIN OLIVE OIL

1 POUND FLANK STEAK, SLICED AGAINST THE GRAIN INTO ½-INCH STRIPS (SEE TIP, PAGE 125)

1 CUP BROCCOLI FLORETS

1 CUP SUGAR SNAP PEAS

1 ZUCCHINI, CHOPPED

¼ CUP STIR-FRY SAUCE (PAGE 149)

1. In a large nonstick skillet over medium-high heat, heat the olive oil until it shimmers.

2. Add the beef and cook 5 to 7 minutes, stirring occasionally, until it browns. Remove with a slotted spoon and set it aside on a platter.

3. Add the broccoli, sugar snap peas, and zucchini. Cook for about 5 minutes, stirring occasionally, until the vegetables are crisp-tender.

4. Return the beef to the pan. Add the stir-fry sauce. Cook for 3 minutes, stirring, until heated through.

PER SERVING Calories: 302; Total Fat: 17g; Total Carbs: 4g; Sugar: 2g; Fiber: 1g; Protein: 33g; Sodium: 523mg

EXTRA-VIRGIN OLIVE OIL

BROCCOLI

GARLIC

GINGER

DAIRY-FREE
GLUTEN-FREE
NUT-FREE
ONE POT

RED BELL PEPPERS

GINGER

GARLIC

DAIRY-FREE
GLUTEN-FREE
NUT-FREE
ONE POT

Beef and Bell Pepper Stir-Fry

SERVES 4 / PREP TIME 5 MINUTES / COOK TIME 10 MINUTES

Lean ground beef cooked with bell peppers, garlic, and ginger is dinner made simple. Serve it with a little soy sauce spooned over some brown rice with steamed veggies on the side for a health-supporting meal that takes only about 15 minutes to prepare.

1 POUND EXTRA-LEAN GROUND BEEF

6 SCALLIONS, WHITE AND GREEN PARTS, CHOPPED

2 RED BELL PEPPERS, CHOPPED

2 TABLESPOONS GRATED FRESH GINGER

½ TEASPOON SEA SALT

3 GARLIC CLOVES, MINCED

1. In a large nonstick skillet over medium-high heat, cook the beef for about 5 minutes, crumbling it with a wooden spoon until it browns.

2. Add the scallions, red bell peppers, ginger, and salt. Cook for about 4 minutes, stirring, until the bell peppers are soft.

3. Add the garlic. Cook for 30 seconds, stirring constantly.

PER SERVING Calories: 599; Total Fat: 19g; Total Carbs: 9g; Sugar: 4g; Fiber: 2g; Protein: 97g; Sodium: 520mg

Beef and Bell Pepper Fajitas

SERVES 4 / PREP TIME 5 MINUTES / COOK TIME 10 MINUTES

Serve these beef strips, bell peppers, and onions with Guacamole (page 48), store-bought salsa, and whole-wheat tortillas for a south-of-the-border treat. You can also use lettuce leaves in place of the tortillas, or use the beef and bell peppers to top a taco salad.

3 TABLESPOONS EXTRA-VIRGIN OLIVE OIL

1½ POUNDS FLANK STEAK, CUT AGAINST THE GRAIN INTO ½-INCH STRIPS (SEE TIP, PAGE 125)

2 GREEN BELL PEPPERS, SLICED

1 ONION, SLICED

1 CUP STORE-BOUGHT SALSA

1 TEASPOON GARLIC POWDER

½ TEASPOON SEA SALT

1. In a large nonstick skillet over medium-high heat, heat the olive oil until it shimmers.

2. Add the beef, bell peppers, and onion. Cook for about 6 minutes, stirring occasionally, until the beef browns.

3. Stir in the salsa, garlic powder, and salt. Cook for 3 minutes, stirring.

PER SERVING Calories: 470; Total Fat: 25g; Total Carbs: 12g; Sugar: 6g; Fiber: 3g; Protein: 49g; Sodium: 722mg

EXTRA-VIRGIN OLIVE OIL

GREEN BELL PEPPERS

TOMATOES

GARLIC

DAIRY-FREE
GLUTEN-FREE
NUT-FREE
ONE POT

Hamburgers with Pub Sauce

SERVES 4 / PREP TIME 10 MINUTES / COOK TIME 10 MINUTES

Burger night has always been popular at my house, and this pub sauce makes hamburgers something special. Top the burgers with your favorite fixings, such as pickles, onion slices, and tomatoes, and serve them on a whole-wheat bun or make lettuce wrap sandwiches.

EXTRA-VIRGIN OLIVE OIL

GARLIC

DAIRY-FREE
NUT-FREE

1 POUND EXTRA-LEAN GROUND BEEF, FORMED INTO 4 PATTIES

½ TEASPOON SEA SALT

⅛ TEASPOON FRESHLY GROUND BLACK PEPPER

½ CUP GARLIC AIOLI (PAGE 151)

3 TABLESPOONS LOW-SODIUM SOY SAUCE

2 TABLESPOONS BROWN SUGAR

2 TABLESPOONS CHOPPED FRESH CHIVES

1. Season the patties with the salt and pepper.

2. In a large skillet over medium-high heat, cook the patties for about 5 minutes per side, or until they register an internal temperature of 145°F on an instant-read meat thermometer.

3. While the hamburgers cook, in a small bowl, whisk the aioli, soy sauce, brown sugar, and chives.

4. Serve the aioli on top of the hamburgers—and anything else that tickles your taste buds.

PER SERVING Calories: 333; Total Fat: 18g; Total Carbs: 13g; Sugar: 7g; Fiber: <1g; Protein: 31g; Sodium: 968mg

Beefy Lentil and Tomato Stew

SERVES 4 / PREP TIME 10 MINUTES / COOK TIME 10 MINUTES

Lentils and tomatoes blend nicely in this simple one-pot stew. Depending on your taste, change up the herbs and spices. Rosemary is good with lentils, as is thyme.

2 TABLESPOONS EXTRA-VIRGIN OLIVE OIL

1 POUND EXTRA-LEAN GROUND BEEF

1 ONION, CHOPPED

1 (14-OUNCE) CAN LENTILS, DRAINED

1 (14-OUNCE) CAN CHOPPED TOMATOES WITH GARLIC AND BASIL, DRAINED

½ TEASPOON SEA SALT

⅛ TEASPOON FRESHLY GROUND BLACK PEPPER

1. In a large pot over medium-high heat, heat the olive oil until it shimmers.

2. Add the beef and onion. Cook for about 5 minutes, crumbling the beef with a wooden spoon until it browns.

3. Stir in the lentils, tomatoes, salt, and pepper. Bring to a simmer. Reduce the heat to medium. Cook for 3 to 4 minutes, stirring, until the lentils are hot.

PER SERVING Calories: 461; Total Fat: 15g; Total Carbs: 37g; Sugar: 2g; Fiber: 17g; Protein: 44g; Sodium: 321mg

EXTRA-VIRGIN OLIVE OIL

TOMATOES

GARLIC

DAIRY-FREE
GLUTEN-FREE
NUT-FREE
ONE POT

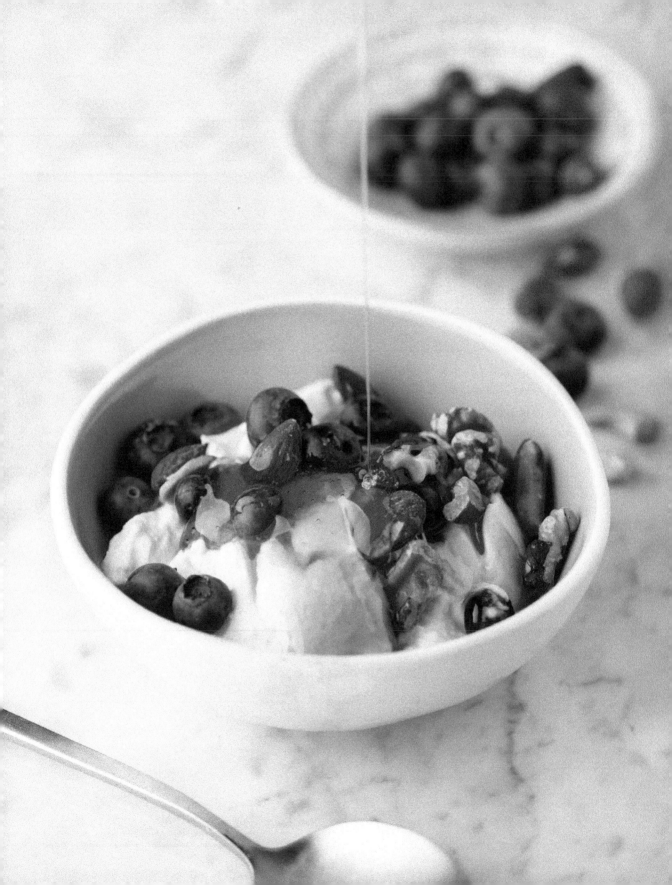

9

DESSERTS

<< Greek Yogurt with Blueberries, Nuts, and Honey, page 138

PECANS

CINNAMON

GLUTEN-FREE
VEGETARIAN

Sweet Spiced Pecans

SERVES 4 / PREP TIME 4 MINUTES / COOK TIME 17 MINUTES

Sweet spiced nuts make a simple yet special dessert. Also try them sprinkled over fruit desserts, such as Honeyed Apple Cinnamon Compote (page 135). They are good warm or cool and keep well in a resealable bag for up to two weeks.

1 CUP PECAN HALVES

¼ CUP PACKED BROWN SUGAR

3 TABLESPOONS UNSALTED BUTTER, MELTED

1 TEASPOON GROUND CINNAMON

½ TEASPOON GROUND NUTMEG

¼ TEASPOON SEA SALT

1. Preheat the oven to 350°F.

2. Line a rimmed baking sheet with parchment paper.

3. In a medium bowl, toss together the pecans, brown sugar, butter, cinnamon, nutmeg, and salt to combine. Spread the nuts in a single layer on the prepared sheet.

4. Bake for 15 to 17 minutes until the nuts are fragrant.

INGREDIENT TIP: You may notice when I use butter or broth in recipes, I always specify unsalted. I do this not because of sodium content, but because it lets you control the amount of salt that goes into your food and adjust it to your taste.

PER SERVING Calories: 323; Total Fat: 30g; Total Carbs: 14g; Sugar: 10g; Fiber: 4g; Protein: 3g; Sodium: 181mg

THE EASY ANTI-INFLAMMATORY DIET

Honeyed Apple Cinnamon Compote

SERVES 4 / PREP TIME 15 MINUTES / COOK TIME 10 MINUTES

Perhaps it's because I live in Washington State, which is known for its apples, but I adore warm apple desserts. These desserts are especially delectable in the fall when apples are in season. Serve this with a scoop of your favorite low-fat vanilla ice cream, or sprinkle it with Sweet Spiced Pecans (page 134) for a crunchy variation. Or enjoy it alone, because it's that good.

6 APPLES, PEELED, CORED, AND CHOPPED

¼ CUP APPLE JUICE

¼ CUP HONEY

1 TEASPOON GROUND CINNAMON

PINCH SEA SALT

In a large pot over medium-high heat, combine the apples, apple juice, honey, cinnamon, and salt. Simmer for about 10 minutes, stirring occasionally, until the apples are still quite chunky but also saucy.

INGREDIENT TIP: I like to experiment with different varieties of apples in compotes to find the right balance of flavors and texture. For this compote I use apples that are a bit on the firm side and quite tart, such as Pink Lady or Braeburn, or a combination.

PER SERVING Calories: 247; Total Fat: <1g; Total Carbs: 66g; Sugar: 54g; Fiber: 9g; Protein: 1g; Sodium: 63mg

CINNAMON

DAIRY-FREE
GLUTEN-FREE
NUT-FREE
ONE POT
VEGETARIAN

GINGER

DAIRY-FREE
GLUTEN-FREE
NUT-FREE
ONE POT
VEGETARIAN

Cranberry Compote

SERVES 4 / PREP TIME 5 MINUTES / COOK TIME 15 MINUTES

Serve this compote warm or chilled. You can eat it by itself, sprinkle it with nuts, use it to dress up plain yogurt or dazzle a piece of pork, or serve it with a scoop of your favorite low-fat vanilla ice cream. With so many possibilities, what are you waiting for?

4 CUPS FRESH CRANBERRIES

¼ CUP HONEY

1 TABLESPOON GRATED FRESH GINGER

JUICE OF 2 ORANGES

ZEST OF 1 ORANGE

In a large pot over medium-high heat, stir together the cranberries, honey, ginger, orange juice, and orange zest. Bring to a boil. Cook for about 10 minutes, stirring occasionally, until the cranberries begin to pop and form a sauce. Chill or serve immediately.

PER SERVING Calories: 172; Total Fat: <1g; Total Carbs: 39g; Sugar: 30g; Fiber: 6g; Protein: 1g; Sodium: 1mg

Coconut Rice with Blueberries

SERVES 4 / PREP TIME 15 MINUTES / COOK TIME 10 MINUTES

Because I have promised quick and easy recipes, rice pudding is out of the question. However, you can make something with similar flavors using precooked brown rice. While I typically recommend lite coconut milk, in this case you'll want the full-fat variety because it is thick and binds the rice a bit better.

1 (14-OUNCE) CAN FULL-FAT
COCONUT MILK

1 CUP FRESH BLUEBERRIES

¼ CUP SUGAR

1 TEASPOON GROUND GINGER

PINCH SEA SALT

2 CUPS COOKED BROWN RICE

1. In a large pot over medium-high heat, combine the coconut milk, blueberries, sugar, ginger, and salt. Cook for about 7 minutes, stirring constantly, until the blueberries soften.

2. Stir in the rice. Cook for about 3 minutes, stirring, until the rice is heated through.

PER SERVING Calories: 469; Total Fat: 25g; Total Carbs: 60g; Sugar: 19g; Fiber: 5g; Protein: 6g; Sodium: 76mg

BLUEBERRIES

GINGER

DAIRY-FREE
GLUTEN-FREE
VEGAN

BLUEBERRIES

MIXED NUTS

GLUTEN-FREE

ONE POT

VEGETARIAN

Greek Yogurt with Blueberries, Nuts, and Honey

SERVES 4 / PREP TIME 5 MINUTES

This is a tasty, quick dessert, and it also makes a delicious breakfast or snack. Feel free to use any nuts that appeal to you, and switch the blueberries for other berries that are seasonally available.

3 CUPS UNSWEETENED PLAIN GREEK YOGURT

1½ CUPS BLUEBERRIES

¾ CUP CHOPPED MIXED NUTS

½ CUP HONEY

Spoon the yogurt into four bowls. Sprinkle with the blueberries and nuts and drizzle with the honey.

PER SERVING Calories: 457; Total Fat: 18g; Total Carbs: 62g; Sugar: 54g; Fiber: 3g; Protein: 15g; Sodium: 213mg

Maple-Glazed Pears with Hazelnuts

SERVES 4 / PREP TIME 10 MINUTES / COOK TIME 20 MINUTES

Pears and hazelnuts do a delicious dance when combined. For this recipe, use pure maple syrup—not the artificially flavored kind made with corn syrup. The payoff is in both flavor and anti-inflammatory goodness.

4 PEARS, PEELED, CORED, AND QUARTERED LENGTHWISE

1 CUP APPLE JUICE

½ CUP PURE MAPLE SYRUP

1 TABLESPOON GRATED FRESH GINGER

¼ CUP CHOPPED HAZELNUTS

1. In a large pot over medium-high heat, combine the pears and apple juice. Bring to a simmer and reduce the heat to medium-low. Cover and simmer for 15 to 20 minutes until the pears soften.

2. While the pears poach, in a small saucepan over medium-high heat, combine the maple syrup and ginger. Bring to a simmer, stirring. Remove the pan from the heat and let the syrup rest.

3. Using a slotted spoon, remove the pears from the poaching liquid and brush with the maple syrup. Serve topped with the hazelnuts.

INGREDIENT TIP: Bosc and Anjou pears are great choices because they are available in most grocery stores and won't fall apart when cooked. However, if there's another interesting variety available, give it a try.

PER SERVING Calories: 286; Total Fat: 3g; Total Carbs: 67g; Sugar: 50g; Fiber: 7g; Protein: 2g; Sodium: 9mg

GINGER

HAZELNUTS

DAIRY-FREE
GLUTEN-FREE
VEGAN

Green Tea–Poached Pears

GREEN TEA

GINGER

DAIRY-FREE
GLUTEN-FREE
NUT-FREE
ONE POT
VEGETARIAN

SERVES 4 / PREP TIME 5 MINUTES / COOK TIME 15 MINUTES

Delicately flavored green tea, ginger, and honey make a beautiful poaching liquid for these flavorful pears. Feel free to add your own spices as well. Consider adding star anise, cinnamon sticks, or whole cloves to the poaching liquid for even more flavor.

4 PEARS, PEELED, CORED, AND QUARTERED LENGTHWISE

2 CUPS STRONGLY BREWED GREEN TEA

¼ CUP HONEY

1 TABLESPOON GRATED FRESH GINGER

In a large pot over medium-high heat, combine the pears, tea, honey, and ginger. Bring to a simmer. Reduce the heat to medium-low, cover, and simmer for about 15 minutes until the pears soften. Serve the pears with the poaching liquid spooned over the top.

PER SERVING Calories: 190; Total Fat: <1g; Total Carbs: 50g; Sugar: 38g; Fiber: 7g; Protein: <1g; Sodium: 4mg

Blueberry Ambrosia

SERVES 4 / PREP TIME 15 MINUTES

Ambrosia salad frequently shows up at potlucks—a combination of fruits with whipped topping mixed in. This anti-inflammatory version has a great combination of soft and crisp fruits and uses coconut milk in place of whipped cream. Toss the can of full-fat coconut milk in the fridge as soon as you get home from the grocery store. That gives it the perfect thickness for this salad.

1 (14-OUNCE) CAN FULL-FAT COCONUT MILK, CHILLED

2 TABLESPOONS HONEY

1 PINT FRESH BLUEBERRIES

1 PINT FRESH RASPBERRIES

1 APPLE, PEELED, CORED, AND CHOPPED

1. Open the chilled can of coconut milk and scoop the solids that have collected on top into a large bowl. Discard any water.

2. Whisk the coconut milk with the honey.

3. Gently stir in the blueberries, raspberries, and apple to coat the fruit with the coconut milk.

SUBSTITUTION TIP: The great thing about this dessert is you can use any fruits you prefer or that are in season. Try oranges, sliced bananas, chopped pears, peaches, nectarines, grapes, or melons.

PER SERVING Calories: 387; Total Fat: 21g; Total Carbs: 46g; Sugar: 31g; Fiber: 11g; Protein: 4g; Sodium: 17mg

BLUEBERRIES

DAIRY-FREE
GLUTEN-FREE
ONE POT
VEGETARIAN

PEANUT BUTTER

GLUTEN-FREE
VEGETARIAN

Easy Peanut Butter Balls

SERVES 15 / PREP TIME 15 MINUTES

While I'm not much of a sweets or dessert eater, I admit to occasionally craving the combination of chocolate and peanut butter. They were clearly made to go together, and these peanut butter balls are the perfect combination of both—and they're ready to eat instantly. No more craving!

¾ CUP CREAMY PEANUT BUTTER

2 TABLESPOONS UNSALTED BUTTER, SOFTENED

1¾ CUPS POWDERED SUGAR

¼ CUP UNSWEETENED COCOA POWDER

½ TEASPOON VANILLA EXTRACT

1. In a medium bowl, stir together the peanut butter, butter, powdered sugar, cocoa powder, and vanilla until well combined.

2. Roll the mixture into about 15 (1-inch) balls and place them on a parchment paper-lined tray. Chill or serve immediately.

STORAGE TIP: These freeze well. Store them frozen in resealable bags for up to 6 months, or keep refrigerated for up to 1 week.

PER SERVING (1 BALL) Calories: 147; Total Fat: 8g; Total Carbs: 17g; Sugar: 15g; Fiber: 1g; Protein: 4g; Sodium: 71mg

Chocolate–Almond Butter Mousse

SERVES 4 / PREP TIME 15 MINUTES

After I discovered my dairy allergy, I stumbled on this mousse when I was trying to come up with a nondairy replacement for pudding. I was thrilled to discover avocado makes a great mousse base. It's creamy and smooth, so it's a perfect backdrop for other flavors.

2 AVOCADOS, PEELED AND PITTED

¼ CUP ALMOND BUTTER

¼ CUP LITE COCONUT MILK

¼ CUP UNSWEETENED COCOA POWDER

¼ CUP PURE MAPLE SYRUP

PINCH SEA SALT

In a blender or food processor, combine the avocados, almond butter, coconut milk, cocoa powder, maple syrup, and salt. Process until smooth.

PER SERVING Calories: 271; Total Fat: 21g; Total Carbs: 23g; Sugar: 12g; Fiber: 7g; Protein: 2g; Sodium: 70mg

ALMOND BUTTER

DAIRY-FREE
GLUTEN-FREE
ONE POT
VEGAN

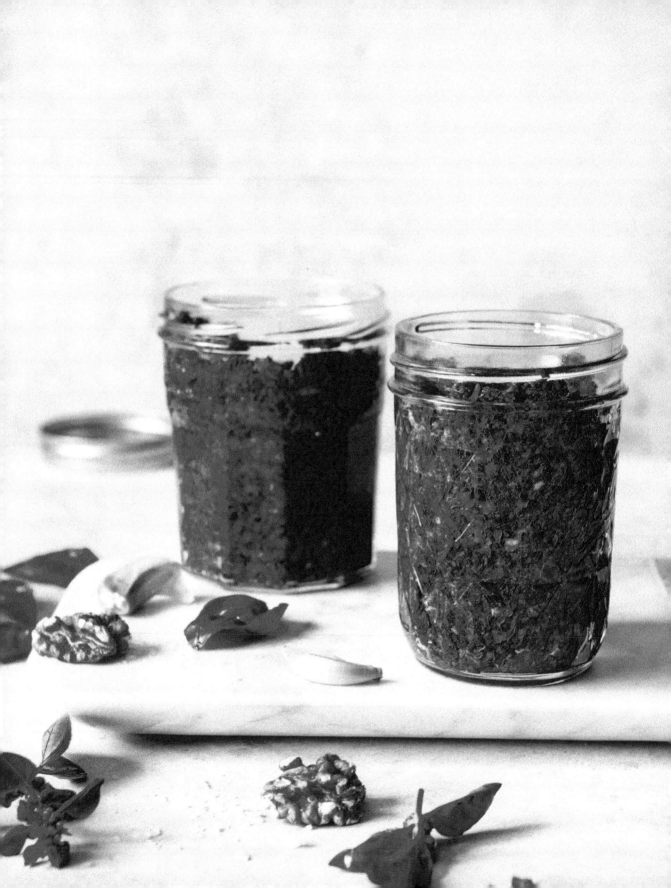

10

SAUCES, CONDIMENTS & DRESSINGS

‹‹ Walnut Pesto, page 146

WALNUTS

EXTRA-VIRGIN OLIVE OIL

GARLIC

SPINACH

GLUTEN-FREE

ONE POT

VEGAN

Walnut Pesto

SERVES 8 / PREP TIME 10 MINUTES

Pesto is a classic pasta topping, tastes delicious on meat or fish (try it on salmon!), and is a delicious spread for flatbreads. This version is vegan because it contains no cheese, which is traditional in pesto.

½ CUP WALNUTS

¼ CUP EXTRA-VIRGIN OLIVE OIL

4 GARLIC CLOVES, MINCED

1 CUP BABY SPINACH

¼ CUP BASIL LEAVES

½ TEASPOON SEA SALT

In a blender or food processor, combine the walnuts, olive oil, garlic, spinach, basil, and salt. Pulse for 15 to 20 (1-second) bursts, or until everything is finely chopped.

PER SERVING Calories: 106; Total Fat: 11g; Total Carbs: 1g; Sugar: <1g; Fiber: <1g; Protein: 2g; Sodium: 120mg

Spinach Pesto

SERVES 4 / PREP TIME 10 MINUTES

Pesto is a handy ingredient. Use it as a pasta sauce, top veggies with it, spread it on a sandwich, or spoon it over meat. You can even marinade seafood in it. This bright green version ups the nutritional content with spinach.

1 CUP FRESH BABY SPINACH

½ CUP FRESH BASIL LEAVES

¼ CUP PINE NUTS

¼ CUP EXTRA-VIRGIN OLIVE OIL

4 GARLIC CLOVES, MINCED

2 OUNCES PARMESAN CHEESE, GRATED

½ TEASPOON SEA SALT

In a blender or food processor, combine the spinach, basil, pine nuts, olive oil, garlic, Parmesan cheese, and salt. Pulse for 15 to 20 (1-second) bursts, or until everything is finely chopped. This keeps refrigerated in a tightly sealed container for 5 days.

SUBSTITUTION TIP: To make this vegan and/or dairy free, omit the Parmesan cheese. If you'd like a cheesy taste anyway, add ¼ cup nutritional yeast.

PER SERVING Calories: 218; Total Fat: 22g; Total Carbs: 3g; Sugar: <1g; Fiber: <1g; Protein: 6g; Sodium: 372mg

SPINACH

EXTRA-VIRGIN
OLIVE OIL

GARLIC

GLUTEN-FREE
ONE POT
VEGETARIAN

EXTRA-VIRGIN
OLIVE OIL

DAIRY-FREE
GLUTEN-FREE
NUT-FREE
ONE POT
VEGETARIAN

Anti-Inflammatory Mayonnaise

MAKES 1 CUP / PREP TIME 10 MINUTES

Making your own mayonnaise is a breeze if you have a blender or food processor, and so much better for you. If you're concerned about the raw egg yolk here, use pasteurized eggs.

1 EGG YOLK

1 TABLESPOON APPLE CIDER VINEGAR

½ TEASPOON DIJON MUSTARD

PINCH SEA SALT

¾ CUP EXTRA-VIRGIN OLIVE OIL

1. In a blender or food processor, combine the egg yolk, cider vinegar, mustard, and salt.

2. Turn on the blender or food processor and while it's running, remove the top spout. Carefully, working one drip at a time to start, drip in the olive oil. After about 15 drops, continue to run the processor and add the oil in a thin stream until emulsified. You may adjust the amount of oil to adjust the thickness. The more oil you add, the thicker the mayonnaise will be.

3. Keep this refrigerated for up to 4 days in a tightly sealed container.

INGREDIENT TIP: It's best to use a neutral flavor of olive oil here. I like the California Olive Ranch Everyday extra-virgin olive oil, which is readily available at most supermarkets.

PER SERVING (2 TABLESPOONS) Calories: 169; Total Fat: 20g; Total Carbs: <1g; Sugar: 0g; Fiber: 0g; Protein: <1g; Sodium: 36mg

Stir-Fry Sauce

SERVES 4 / PREP TIME 5 MINUTES

Stir-fry sauce in the flick of a whisk! But before you add it to any stir-fry, whisk it again to incorporate the arrowroot powder and add it to the hot pan. It brings a lot of flavor. Choose a low-sodium soy sauce or if you need a gluten-free option, choose gluten-free soy sauce or tamari.

¼ CUP LOW-SODIUM SOY SAUCE

3 GARLIC CLOVES, MINCED

JUICE OF 2 LIMES

1 TABLESPOON GRATED FRESH GINGER

1 TABLESPOON ARROWROOT POWDER

In a small bowl, whisk together the soy sauce, garlic, lime juice, ginger, and arrowroot powder.

INGREDIENT TIP: Arrowroot powder is a thickener similar to cornstarch. You can find it online or at health food stores. If you can't find it, don't worry. Just use cornstarch.

PER SERVING (2 TABLESPOONS) Calories: 24; Total Fat: 0g; Total Carbs: 4g; Sugar: 2g; Fiber: 0g; Protein: 1g; Sodium: 887mg

GARLIC

GINGER

DAIRY-FREE
NUT-FREE
ONE POT
VEGAN

GINGER

GARLIC

DAIRY-FREE
NUT-FREE
ONE POT
VEGAN

Ginger-Teriyaki Sauce

SERVES 4 / PREP TIME 5 MINUTES

Sweet and savory teriyaki sauce is really good on meat, poultry, and fish. I even like it warmed and drizzled over brown rice. A few recipes in this book use this sauce, which comes together in an instant.

¼ CUP LOW-SODIUM SOY SAUCE

¼ CUP PINEAPPLE JUICE

2 TABLESPOONS PACKED BROWN SUGAR

1 TABLESPOON GRATED FRESH GINGER

1 TABLESPOON ARROWROOT POWDER OR CORNSTARCH

1 TEASPOON GARLIC POWDER

In a small bowl, whisk the soy sauce, pineapple juice, brown sugar, ginger, arrowroot powder, and garlic powder. Keep refrigerated in a tightly sealed container for up to 5 days.

SUBSTITUTION TIP: For a gluten-free version, use gluten-free soy sauce or tamari.

PER SERVING (ABOUT 2 TABLESPOONS) Calories: 41; Total Fat: 0g; Total Carbs: 10g; Sugar: 7g; Fiber: 0g; Protein: 1g; Sodium: 882mg

Garlic Aioli

SERVES 4 / PREP TIME 5 MINUTES

Aioli is just a fancy name for a flavored mayonnaise, typically with garlic. This recipe uses Anti-Inflammatory Mayonnaise (page 148) as the base. Customize this recipe with flavors you enjoy. Some other flavored mayos I like to make include Sriracha mayonnaise (1 tablespoon Sriracha to ½ cup mayo) and citrus mayonnaise (with the zest of 1 citrus fruit stirred into the mayo).

½ CUP ANTI-INFLAMMATORY MAYONNAISE (PAGE 148)

3 GARLIC CLOVES, FINELY MINCED

In a small bowl, whisk the mayonnaise and garlic to combine. Keep refrigerated in a tightly sealed container for up to 4 days.

VARIATION TIP: For red pepper aioli, add 3 slices store-bought roasted red pepper to the mayo and process for another 60 seconds after it is done.

PREPARATION TIP: This recipe makes investing in a garlic press worthwhile. The garlic press gives you finely minced garlic without any big chunks (something you can also do with a knife). To mince garlic as small as possible without a garlic press, place the flat side of the knife blade on a peeled garlic clove and carefully smash down on the flat of the blade with your hand. It will crush the clove. From there, chop it finely.

PER SERVING (2 TABLESPOONS) Calories: 169; Total Fat: 20g; Total Carbs: <1g; Sugar: 0g; Fiber: 0g; Protein: <1g; Sodium: 36mg

EXTRA-VIRGIN OLIVE OIL

GARLIC

DAIRY-FREE
GLUTEN-FREE
NUT-FREE
ONE POT
VEGETARIAN

**EXTRA-VIRGIN
OLIVE OIL**

GARLIC

DAIRY-FREE
GLUTEN-FREE
NUT-FREE
ONE POT
VEGAN

Raspberry Vinaigrette

SERVES 8 / PREP TIME 5 MINUTES

Top a salad with this dressing, toss it with veggies, or use it as a marinade for fish or seafood. This vinaigrette can transform any food with its bright flavors. The raspberries have a nice acidity and bring a lot of flavor to dishes. This will keep refrigerated for up to five days. However, if you do refrigerate it, the olive oil will solidify, so set it out on the counter for 30 to 45 minutes before you use it.

¾ CUP EXTRA-VIRGIN OLIVE OIL

¼ CUP APPLE CIDER VINEGAR

¼ CUP FRESH RASPBERRIES, CRUSHED
WITH THE BACK OF A SPOON

3 GARLIC CLOVES, FINELY MINCED

½ TEASPOON SEA SALT

⅛ TEASPOON FRESHLY GROUND
BLACK PEPPER

In a small bowl, whisk the olive oil, cider vinegar, raspberries, garlic, salt, and pepper. Keep refrigerated in a tightly sealed container for up to 5 days.

PER SERVING (ABOUT 2 TABLESPOONS) Calories: 167; Total Fat: 19g; Total Carbs: <1g; Sugar: 0g; Fiber: 0g; Protein: <1g; Sodium: 118mg

Lemon-Ginger Vinaigrette

SERVES 8 / PREP TIME 5 MINUTES

Vinaigrettes are excellent for doing double duty as dressings and marinades, and this one is no exception. It's a zesty pork marinade, and equally good on tossed salads or even used as a coleslaw dressing with shredded cabbage (one of my favorites).

¾ CUP EXTRA-VIRGIN OLIVE OIL

¼ CUP FRESHLY SQUEEZED
LEMON JUICE

1 TABLESPOON GRATED FRESH GINGER

1 GARLIC CLOVE, MINCED

½ TEASPOON SEA SALT

⅛ TEASPOON FRESHLY GROUND
BLACK PEPPER

In a small bowl, whisk the olive oil, lemon juice, ginger, garlic, salt, and pepper. Keep refrigerated in a tightly sealed container for up to 5 days.

PER SERVING (2 TABLESPOONS) Calories: 167; Total Fat: 19g; Total Carbs: <1g; Sugar: 0g; Fiber: 0g; Protein: <1g; Sodium: 118mg

EXTRA-VIRGIN
OLIVE OIL

GINGER

DAIRY-FREE
GLUTEN-FREE
NUT-FREE
ONE POT
VEGAN

PEANUT BUTTER

GARLIC

GINGER

DAIRY-FREE
ONE POT
VEGAN

Peanut Sauce

SERVES 8 / PREP TIME 5 MINUTES

I have been a fan of peanut sauce since my very first taste, and I'm always whipping up new versions. If you like a spicier sauce, add 1 tablespoon Sriracha sauce. Otherwise, enjoy it as is; it's still really good.

1 CUP LITE COCONUT MILK

¼ CUP CREAMY PEANUT BUTTER

¼ CUP FRESHLY SQUEEZED LIME JUICE

3 GARLIC CLOVES, MINCED

2 TABLESPOONS LOW-SODIUM SOY SAUCE, OR GLUTEN-FREE SOY SAUCE, OR TAMARI

1 TABLESPOON GRATED FRESH GINGER

In a blender or food processor, process the coconut milk, peanut butter, lime juice, garlic, soy sauce, and ginger until smooth. Keep refrigerated in a tightly sealed container for up to 5 days.

PER SERVING (ABOUT 2 TABLESPOONS) Calories: 143; Total Fat: 11g; Total Carbs: 8g; Sugar: 2g; Fiber: 1g; Protein: 6g; Sodium: 533mg

Garlic Ranch Dressing

SERVES 8 / PREP TIME 5 MINUTES

This Greek yogurt ranch dressing is a perfect sandwich spread, as well as an excellent topper for salads or as a dip for vegetables. You can also substitute cottage cheese for nonfat plain Greek yogurt, or use half cottage cheese and half yogurt.

1 CUP NONFAT PLAIN GREEK YOGURT

1 GARLIC CLOVE, MINCED

2 TABLESPOONS CHOPPED, FRESH CHIVES

¼ CUP CHOPPED, FRESH DILL

ZEST OF 1 LEMON

½ TEASPOON SEA SALT

⅛ TEASPOON FRESHLY CRACKED BLACK PEPPER

In a small bowl, whisk together the yogurt, garlic, chives, dill, lemon zest, salt, and pepper. Keep refrigerated in a tightly sealed container for up to 5 days.

PER SERVING Calories: 17, Total Fat: 0g; Total Carbs: 3g; Sugar: 2g; Fiber: 0g; Protein: 2g; Sodium: 140mg

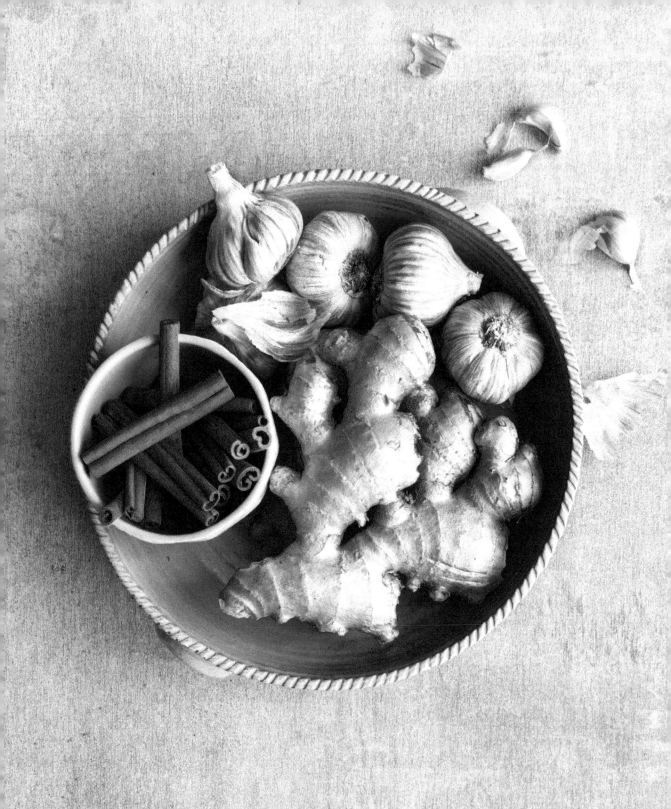

The Dirty Dozen & the Clean Fifteen

A nonprofit and environmental watchdog organization called the Environmental Working Group (EWG) looks at data supplied by the U.S. Department of Agriculture (USDA) and the Food and Drug Administration (FDA) about pesticide residues. Each year it compiles a list of the lowest and highest pesticide loads found in commercial crops. You can use these lists to decide which fruits and vegetables to buy organic to minimize your exposure to pesticides and which produce is considered safe enough to buy conventionally. This does not mean they are pesticide-free, though, so wash these fruits and vegetables thoroughly.

THE DIRTY DOZEN

- » Apples
- » Celery
- » Cherry tomatoes
- » Cucumbers
- » Grapes
- » Nectarines (imported)
- » Peaches
- » Potatoes
- » Snap peas (imported)
- » Spinach
- » Strawberries
- » Sweet bell peppers

Kale/Collard greens & Hot peppers*

THE CLEAN FIFTEEN

- » Asparagus
- » Avocados
- » Cabbage
- » Cantaloupes (domestic)
- » Cauliflower
- » Eggplants
- » Grapefruits
- » Kiwis
- » Mangoes
- » Onions
- » Papayas
- » Pineapples
- » Sweet corn
- » Sweet peas (frozen)
- » Sweet potatoes

*In addition to the Dirty Dozen, the EWG added two produce items contaminated with highly toxic organophosphate insecticides.

Measurement Conversions

VOLUME EQUIVALENTS (LIQUID)

US STANDARD	US STANDARD (OUNCES)	METRIC (APPROXIMATE)
2 tablespoons	1 fl. oz.	30 mL
¼ cup	2 fl. oz.	60 mL
½ cup	4 fl. oz.	120 mL
1 cup	8 fl. oz.	240 mL
1½ cups	12 fl. oz.	355 mL
2 cups or 1 pint	16 fl. oz.	475 mL
4 cups or 1 quart	32 fl. oz.	1 L
1 gallon	128 fl. oz.	4 L

OVEN TEMPERATURES

FAHRENHEIT (F)	CELSIUS (C) (APPROXIMATE)
250°F	120°C
300°F	150°C
325°F	165°C
350°F	180°C
375°F	190°C
400°F	200°C
425°F	220°C
450°F	230°C

VOLUME EQUIVALENTS (DRY)

US STANDARD	METRIC (APPROXIMATE)
⅛ teaspoon	0.5 mL
¼ teaspoon	1 mL
½ teaspoon	2 mL
¾ teaspoon	4 mL
1 teaspoon	5 mL
1 tablespoon	15 mL
¼ cup	59 mL
⅓ cup	79 mL
½ cup	118 mL
⅔ cup	156 mL
¾ cup	177 mL
1 cup	235 mL
2 cups or 1 pint	475 mL
3 cups	700 mL
4 cups or 1 quart	1 L
½ gallon	2 L
1 gallon	4 L

WEIGHT EQUIVALENTS

US STANDARD	METRIC (APPROXIMATE)
½ ounce	15 g
1 ounce	30 g
2 ounces	60 g
4 ounces	115 g
8 ounces	225 g
12 ounces	340 g
16 ounces or 1 pound	455 g

Resources

Shopping

Amazon.com has any ingredient you could possibly want, shipped to you quickly. It's where I get my arrowroot powder with the click of a mouse, without leaving the house, my garlic press, and the rasp-style grater I use for grating fresh ginger. They are both made by Zyliss.

Websites

Dr. Andrew Weil has great recommendations for an anti-inflammatory diet: www.drweil.com /health-wellness/health-centers/aging-gracefully/dr-weils-anti-inflammatory-diet/.

Dr. Barry Sears is an expert on anti-inflammatory nutrition. Visit his website at www.DrSears.com.

Since research is linking heart disease to inflammation, the American Heart Association certainly has something to say about it. Visit www.heart.org.

The American Autoimmune Related Diseases Association offers excellent resources for people with inflammatory conditions. Visit www.AARDA.org.

The Arthritis Foundation is a big proponent of the anti-inflammatory diet because inflammation is such a key part of arthritis. Visit www.arthritis.org

The Mediterranean Diet is an outstanding anti-inflammatory diet. Learn more at www.MediterraneanDiet.com.

Books

If you want more anti-inflammatory recipes, consider these books:

Blum, Susan, MD, MPH. *The Immune System Recovery Plan*. New York: Scribner, 2013.

Bruner, Sondi. *Anti-Inflammatory Diet in 21*. Berkeley, CA: Rockridge Press, 2015.

Calimeris, Dorothy. *The Anti-Inflammatory Diet & Action Plans.* Berkeley, CA: Sonoma Press, 2015.

Given, Madeline, NC, and Jennifer Langs MD. *The Anti-Inflammatory Diet Cookbook: No-Hassle 30-Minute Recipes to Reduce Inflammation.* Berkeley, CA: Rockridge Press, 2017.

The Mediterranean Diet for Beginners. Berkeley, CA: Rockridge Press, 2013.

The Mediterranean Slow Cooker Cookbook. Berkeley, CA: Salinas Press, 2014.

Zogheib, Susan. *The Mediterranean Diet Plan: Heart-Healthy Recipes & Meal Plans for Every Type of Eater.* Berkeley, CA: Rockridge Press, 2016.

Here are two books I have written about Hashimoto's disease:

Frazier, Karen. *The Hashimoto's Cookbook and Action Plan: 31 Days to Eliminate Toxins and Restore Thyroid Health through Diet.* Berkeley, CA: Rockridge Press, 2015.

———. *The Hashimoto's 4-Week Plan: A Holistic Guide to Treating Hypothyroidism.* Berkeley, CA: Sonoma Press, 2016.

References

American Autoimmune Related Diseases Association. "List of Autoimmune Diseases." Accessed March 30, 2017. www.aarda.org/disease-list/.

American College of Rheumatology. "NSAIDs (Nonsteroidal Anti-Inflammatory Drugs)." Accessed March 30, 2017. www.rheumatology.org/I-Am-A/Patient-Caregiver /Treatments/NSAIDs.

American Heart Association. "Inflammation and Heart Disease." Last modified October 12, 2016. Accessed March 30, 2017. www.heart.org/HEARTORG/Conditions /Inflammation-and-Heart-Disease_UCM_432150_Article.jsp#.WM62KxIrJxh.

Arthritis Foundation. "8 Food Ingredients that Can Cause Inflammation." *ArthritisToday*. Accessed December 30, 2016. www.arthritis.org/living-with-arthritis/arthritis-diet /foods-to-avoid-limit/food-ingredients-and-inflammation-2.php.

Arthritis Foundation. "Add These Arthritis-Friendly Foods to Your Diet." *Living with Arthritis Blog*. August 13, 2015. Accessed March 30, 2017. blog.arthritis.org/living-with-arthritis /arthritis-friendly-foods/.

Arthritis Foundation. "Health Benefits of Ginger for Arthritis." *Living with Arthritis Blog*. January 2016. Accessed March 30, 2017. blog.arthritis.org/living-with-arthritis /health-benefits-of-ginger/.

Arthritis Foundation. "Olive Oil Reduces Arthritis Inflammation." *Living with Arthritis Blog*. January 25, 2016. Accessed March 30, 2017. blog.arthritis.org/living-with-arthritis /olive-oil-anti-inflammatory-arthritis-diet/.

Beyond Celiac. "Non-Celiac Gluten Sensitivity." Accessed March 2017. www.beyondceliac.org /celiac-disease/non-celiac-gluten-sensitivity/.

Chao, L. K., K. F. Hua, H. Y. Hsu, S. S. Cheng, I. F. Lin, C. J. Chen, S. T. Chen, and S. T. Chang. "Cinnamaldehyde Inhibits Pro-Inflammatory Cytokines Secretion from Monocytes /Macrophages through Suppression of Intracellular Signaling." *Food and Chemical Toxicology* 46, no. 1 (January 2008): 220–31. doi:10.1016/j.fct.2007.07.016.

da Rosa, J. S., M. B. Facchin, J. Bastos, M. A. Siqueira, G. A. Micke, E. M. Dalmarco, M. G. Pizzolatti, and T. S. Fröde. "Systemic Administration of Rosmarinus Officinalis Attenuates the Inflammatory Response Induced by Carrageenan in the Mouse Model of Pleurisy." *Planta Medica* 79, no. 17 (November 2013): 1605–14. doi:10.1055/s-0033-1351018.

DiCorleto, Paul, PhD. "Why You Should Pay Attention to Chronic Inflammation." *Health Essentials from Cleveland Clinic.* July 25, 2016. Accessed March 30, 2017. health.clevelandclinic.org/2014/10/why-you-should-pay-attention-to-chronic-inflammation/.

Galland, L. "Diet and Inflammation." *Nutrition in Clinical Practice* 25, no. 6 (December 2010): 634–40. doi:10.1177/0884533610385703.

Gupta, Subash C., Sridevi Patchva, and Bharat B. Aggarwal. "Therapeutic Roles of Curcumin: Lessons Learned from Clinical Trials." *The AAPS Journal* 15, no. 1 (January 2013): 195–218. doi:10.1208/s12248-012-9432-8.

Harvard Health Publications. "Foods that Fight Inflammation." Harvard Medical School. June 2014. Last updated October 26, 2015. Accessed March 30, 2017. www.health.harvard.edu/staying-healthy/foods-that-fight-inflammation.

Kresser, Chris. "How Too Much Omega-6 and Not Enough Omega-3 Is Making Us Sick." May 8, 2010. Accessed March 30, 2017. www.chriskresser.com/how-too-much-omega-6-and-not-enough-omega-3-is-making-us-sick/.

Marshall Protocol Knowledge Base. "Incidence and Prevalence of Chronic Disease." Autoimmunity Research Foundation. November 28, 2016. Accessed March 30, 2017. www.mpkb.org/home/pathogenesis/epidemiology.

National Institutes of Health. "Understanding Autoinflammatory Disease." National Institute of Arthritis and Musculoskeletal and Skin Diseases. January 2017. Accessed March 30, 2017. www.niams.nih.gov/health_info/autoinflammatory/.

Nordqvist, Christian. "Inflammation: Causes, Symptoms, and Treatment." *Medical News Today.* Last updated September 16, 2015. Accessed March 2017. www.medicalnewstoday.com/articles/248423.php.

Palozza, P., N. Parrone, A. Catalano, and R. Simone. "Tomato Lycopene and Inflammatory Cascade: Basic Interactions and Clinical Implications." *Current Medicinal Chemistry* 17, no. 21 (2010): 2547–63.

Schäfer, Georgia, and Catherine H. Kaschula. "The Immunomodulation and Anti-Inflammatory Effects of Garlic Organosulfur Compounds in Cancer Chemoprevention." *Anticancer Agents in Medicinal Chemistry* 14, no. 2 (February 2014): 233–240. doi:10.2174/18715206113136660370.

Seliger, Susan. "'Superfoods Everyone Needs." WebMD. Accessed March 30, 2017. www.webmd.com/diet/features/superfoods-everyone-needs#1.

Sun, T., Z. Xu, C. T. Wu, M. Janes, W. Prinyawiwatkul, and H. K. No. "Antioxidant Activities of Different Colored Sweet Bell Peppers (Capsicum Annuum L.)." *Journal of Food Science* 72, no. 2 (March 2007): S98–102. doi:10.1111/j.1750-3841.2006.00245.x.

Taylor & Francis. "Curcumin and Turmeric: Improving the Therapeutic Benefits by Enhancing Absorption and Bioavailability." *ScienceDaily.* August 12, 2015. Accessed March 30, 2017. www.sciencedaily.com/releases/2015/08/150812134254.htm.

University of Maryland Medical Center. "Green Tea." November 6, 2015. Accessed March 30, 2017. http://umm.edu/health/medical/altmed/herb/green-tea.

U.S. National Library of Medicine. "What Is an Inflammation?" Informed Health Online. January 7, 2015. Accessed March 30, 2017. www.ncbi.nlm.nih.gov/pubmedhealth /PMH0072482/.

WebMD. "Steroids to Treat Arthritis." Accessed March 30, 2017. www.webmd.com /rheumatoid-arthritis/guide/steroids-to-treat-arthritis#1.

Weil, Andrew, MD. "Anti-Inflammatory Herbs." DrWeil.com. February 28, 2017. Accessed March 30, 2017. www.drweil.com/vitamins-supplements-herbs/herbs/can-herbs -combat-inflammation/.

Weil, Andrew, MD. "Dr. Weil's Anti Inflammatory Diet." DrWeil.com. Accessed March 30, 2017. www.drweil.com/health-wellness/health-centers/aging-gracefully/dr-weils -anti-inflammatory-diet/.

Wellen, Kathryn E., and Gökhan S. Hotamisligil. "Inflammation, Stress, and Diabetes." *Journal of Clinical Investigation* 115, no. 5 (May 2, 2005): 1111–1119. doi:10.1172/JCI25102.

Recipe Index

Key Ingredient List

Index

About the Author

Karen Frazier is a freelance writer who has written several cookbooks for people on special diets. Previous cookbooks include *The Hashimoto's 4-Week Plan*, *The Acid Reflux Escape Plan*, and *The Hashimoto's Cookbook and Action Plan*, among others. Karen has learned to control her inflammatory conditions, along with multiple food sensitivities, through lifestyle and dietary changes. Karen lives in western Washington near Seattle with her husband and four dogs.

Printed in the USA
CPSIA information can be obtained
at www.ICGtesting.com
CBHW041032060524
8112CB00003B/11